BMA

Practice: Demanding Work

Understanding patterns of work in primary care

John Waller
Health Information Analyst
Centre for Innovation in Primary Care, Sheffield

and

Paul Hodgkin
Previously Co-Director
Centre for Innovation in Primary Care, Sheffield

Radcliffe Medical Press

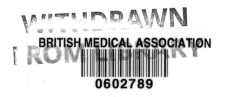

© 2000 John Waller and Paul Hodgkin

Radcliffe Medical Press Ltd
18 Marcham Road, Abingdon, Oxon OX14 1AA

British Library Cataloguing in Publication Data

A catalogue record for this book is available from the British Library.

ISBN 1 85775 447 6

Typeset by Joshua Associates Ltd, Oxford
Printed and bound by TJ International Ltd, Padstow, Cornwall

Contents

Preface

> *Friday 7 pm*
>
> 'There goes the last patient. Once again my hopes for an early finish scuppered by all those emergency extras that just had to be fitted it . . . the end to another demanding week. Our neighbouring practice on Myrtle Road never seems to be this harassed. Maybe they have easier patients? Maybe they restrict the demand by providing a lower quality service? Maybe they are better organised than us or have come up with some innovative appointment system? Maybe they are better at pretending to cope?'
>
> 'So how are you going to find out the answers to all these questions? Perhaps by a practice team visit, perhaps by arranging some shadowing exercises with Myrtle Road? Or how about doing some workload data comparison with them and all the others in the Primary Care Group?'
>
> 'Data comparison – you mean league tables, name and shame and all that?'
>
> 'No, it doesn't have to be done that way. We mean benchmarking, comparing data with your peers that nobody outside of the PCG need see. Discovering where you stand in relation to everybody else, finding out who does things differently, being prepared to learn from others. You might even discover that you are doing an excellent job in really difficult circumstances.'

It feels like a time of rapid change in the way general practice in Britain is organised. Yet on another level its core function – seeing one million patients every working day – remains very stable. This book will help anybody with an interest in the present and future of general practice to better understand how it currently handles that core function, and how it might do it differently in the future. As such, it will be of interest to health service managers, researchers, public health physicians, and PCG/Trust board members. Our principal readership though will be those who work directly in general practice – GPs, nurses, practice managers and receptionists.

This book can be read from cover to cover like any other, but we also see it as a reference book, another in the long line of Radcliffe Medical Press publications that can be there on the practice library shelf ready to be consulted. For a practice team thinking about changing its appointment system, or struggling with a perceived problem with defaulters, we see this book as a place to turn to for some comparative data; some useful tips and some pointers as to who else (as of June 2000) had researched the issue.

The book, in large part, summarises the findings of six years of data comparison and analysis involving up to 33 practices in Sheffield. In most chapters we refer to earlier reports that we have been involved in producing that go into more detail on a particular issue. Individual copies of those reports can be obtained free from:

The Centre for Innovation in Primary Care, Walsh Court, 10 Bells Square, Sheffield S1 2FY. Tel: 0114 220 2000   Fax: 0114 220 2001   Email: cipc@innovate.org.uk

Some of the more recent reports, plus the database toolkit for analysing computer appointment data, can be downloaded from our website:

www.innovate.org.uk

We hope we have written something that helps practices to better understand their workload and thus provide an improved service for their patients. We also hope that it enables them to make the conditions under which they work a little less demanding.

John Waller
Paul Hodgkin
August 2000

Acknowledgements

Many others have contributed to the body of work over six years on which this book is based. In particular, the idea and impetus for the original Practice Data Comparison project came from Rosalind Eve and Jeanette McGorrigan. Special recognition should go to:

- **Rosalind Eve** – now the Director of the Centre for Innovation in Primary Care, and the person who designed and set up the Practice Data Comparison project and directed its work for five years
- **Pete Jenkins** – the original project worker who established the original database and, even more importantly, established the working relationships with the participating practices
- **Jeanette McGorrigan** – the GP whose own interest and work on practice data collection inspired the development of the project.

We would also like to mention and thank:

- **the Sheffield practices** who provided us with this data
- **Karen Kilner** – who worked on the project as a health information analyst for 18 months
- **Kay Noble** – who at various times assisted with the data input
- **Simon Dixon** – the health economist who gave us essential methodological advice for our work on costing consultations
- **Steve Maxwell** – who designed the database for the analysis of computer appointment data
- **Sheffield Health and Trent NHS Executive** for funding the work
- **Gordon Reid**, Director of Sheffield Health's Information Department and his staff for help and collaboration over many years.

And last but definitely not least:

- **the administrative staff** in those practices who for up to six years have been patiently filling in our monthly data sheets.

1 Introduction

In 1999 general practice directly cost the British taxpayer about £3 billion. Prescriptions for drugs cost about a further £4 billion and general practitioners (GPs) referred 11 million patients to hospital with considerable financial consequences for the National Health Service (NHS). In short, general practice is big business. Yet this key public service has hardly been managed in any direct way at all. Instead it is provided by some 30 000 practitioners working in nearly 10 000 practices. These small organisations have typically been under-managed and under-capitalised when compared both to hospital care and to other systems of primary care in the developed world.

For many decades general practitioners in Britain have resembled homesteaders, each tending their own little farm. Neither collaborating nor truly competing with their neighbours, each could do pretty much as they wished. This lack of interest in how colleagues did the job was especially marked in relation to work patterns. Just as farmers discuss the weather or the prices in the market, GPs discussed in an anecdotal way what the workload was like and how the business was going. Hard data was rare. Some practices added up the figures in their appointment books to measure their own workload, most did not, and nobody knew, beyond anecdote, what anybody else was experiencing. Data about individual patients was there in abundance, but buried in handwritten and typed pieces of paper in record envelopes dating from Lloyd George's era.

Imagine yourself as the new chief executive of General Practice plc in, say, 1990. One million people came through your doors every day for a consultation, and your information systems for recording what was happening to them had barely entered the 20th century. General practice was like a black box. Staff, time and money went in, consultations, referrals and prescriptions came out, but very little was known about what was going on inside the box.

The 1990s saw some progress. A growing amount of the work of general practice is now recorded on computer, though using software that is often 10 years behind the times and from many competing companies whose systems rarely communicate with anybody else's. Practices also began to collaborate with each other – to share out-of-hours care in GP cooperatives, and to commission secondary care services in multi-funds, total purchasing pilots or locality commissioning groups.

Times change. The new primary care groups (PCGs) and trusts (PCTs) need to understand and influence the services their practices deliver, ensure that national service frameworks and clinical governance agendas are delivered, and manage resources efficiently and effectively. In short, the Government is out to ensure that patients receive efficient, transparent and consistent care and that general practice is finally brought into the managerial mainstream of the NHS.

The future requires new levels of information and understanding. Some of this will be about clinical effectiveness – what works, what does not, and what is in the enormous grey area where the art of being a GP still holds sway. But information about workload is also crucial. The bread and butter of general practice remains dealing with that million patients every day – those wanting advice or reassurance, wanting an explanation or diagnosis of what is happening to them, wanting a prescription, wanting a referral, wanting a sympathetic ear to listen to their story.

We have experienced that daily demand, one as a practice manager, one as a GP, in different practices, and we know the pressures involved in coping with it. It is indeed demanding work. For ten years, in changing roles, we have been involved in projects in Sheffield to work collaboratively, to share information, to provide measures to benchmark how our practices were doing compared to others, and to use this information for the benefit of the service we provided. The aim has been to improve the quality of the service, and the quality of the working life of those who work within it. But if we are honest it has often been about finding pragmatic coping strategies for dealing with a heavy workload – maintaining the service and maintaining the morale of its workers.

For six years, through the Sheffield Practice Data Comparison (PDC) project, we have been collecting and analysing data on general practice activity rates in Sheffield. The results have been fed back to practices and other interested parties within Sheffield as individual reports. Since 1998 the project has been part of the Centre for Innovation in Primary Care, and some more recent reports have been circulated to every health authority and PCG. This book – *General Practice: Demanding Work* – presents the learning from the project in its totality to a national audience.

Results are presented so that those who work in general practice can compare their own data, if they have it, with our data. We do not claim that the results from 30 practices in one city are typical or represent a statistical average. But in a situation where comparative data is scarce they represent a useful benchmark, a step beyond the black box.

We have tried to make how we arrived at our results transparent, so that others can replicate the analysis on their own data if they wish, but without presenting excessive detail for other readers. For those who want to know more about our results and methodology, they are free to contact us for further information and copies of our reports, or to visit the Centre for Innovation in Primary Care's website (www.innovate.org.uk) and to download material from it.

Benchmarking alone is useful. For a practice to know, for instance, that its default rate on appointments is high, low or average can lead to that practice taking appropriate action. At points in the book, however, we go beyond presenting results to make suggestions about what practices might do to improve their service. We *do not* claim to be the experts in how to run a general practice, if such people exist we have yet to meet them. We *do* think that the work we have done provides a rich source of evidence-based learning on what is really happening in general practice and how it might be done better.

We are, of course, not alone in analysing consultation patterns in general practice. National surveys have been undertaken, and pieces of research have occurred based on data from one or more practices. In most chapters we present a brief section on what others have found, providing information and references for those who want to follow up the issue in more depth.

This is a time of great change for general practice – so much so that there are questions about the future role of the general practitioner itself. Can the self-employed GP principle be flexible enough to survive long into the 21st century? Will a salaried service or nurses replace the general practitioner? To give the title of this book an alternative meaning, do GPs have the right to *demand work*, to demand a job? The data about consultations contained in this book sheds some light on these questions, particularly the relationship between the work that practice nurses do and that of GPs. Questions about the role of the GP itself are addressed, more polemically, in Chapter 20.

GPs and practice nurses spend their days dealing with, and thinking about, unique individual patients. Our focus is on aggregate behaviour – not the one patient in a 100 that stood out, but the 99 who did not. All too often bright ideas for change founder because they are rooted in myths about what is actually happening on the ground. If we enable readers to better understand the daily reality of general practice, perhaps dispelling a few myths along the way, then this book will have been worth writing.

2 Studying consultation patterns

Studying consultation patterns involves a trade-off between:

- *representativeness* – collecting data from a sample that allows generalisations to be drawn about all practices
- *completeness* – covering all aspects of practice work
- *workload* – keeping the work involved to a minimum.

This trade-off has produced two broad approaches.

In the first, enthusiasts design and collect their own data drawn from one or a small number of practices. Much of the literature is of this type and we will be reporting many of its conclusions throughout this book. The drawbacks of this method include non-standardised definitions and dependence on enthusiasts. These make the results less useable to everyday practices or PCGs who wish to understand their patterns of work and make changes.

The second approach is to collect standardised data from large groups of practices or populations of patients. This method is more likely to generate representative results since the sample is both larger and can be recruited in ways that increase representativeness. To the extent that this method can be adapted to use the routine data generated by many computerised systems, it can also form the basis of internal benchmarking for practices and organisations outside the original participants. The Sheffield data used throughout this book falls into this category.

Since such studies form the backdrop for this book, the next section summarises the main national surveys that are useful when studying workload.

The National Morbidity Surveys of England and Wales

The most extensive source of information on general practice workload comes from the decennial National Morbidity Surveys (NMS) of England and Wales, of which there have been four, with the last in 1991/2.

The 1991/2 survey involved 60 volunteer practices in England and Wales who, for a full year, recorded every face-to-face contact with patients who were on the practices' age–sex registers – over 500 000 patients in all. Socio-economic data was also recorded by questionnaire for 83% of the patients. Comparison with the 1991 census showed that the patients were representative of the general population. The practices were geographically diverse, but tended to be larger than average with younger GPs and more ancillary staff. They also had to be amongst the 34% of general practices that at that time had the necessary computer system to record details of every consultation.

The principal purpose of the survey was to provide epidemiological data on *morbidity*. The reason(s) for every face-to-face contact with a doctor or practice nurse, either in the surgery or the patient's home, was recorded, thus providing a wealth of data on the prevalence and incidence of disease. However, as a by-product the survey also provided an extensive record of *workload* and the determinants of it.

We present in Appendix 1 four key graphs on contact rates from the survey. These are reproduced by kind permission of the authors. The full report is:

McCormick A, Fleming D and Charlton J (1995) *Morbidity Statistics from General Practice: fourth national study 1991–1992.* A study carried out by the Royal College of General Practitioners, the Office of Population Censuses and Surveys, and the Department of Health. HMSO, London.

Amongst the key workload, conclusions of the survey were:

- broadly 'J'-shaped curves for age-specific contact rates with doctors and nurses in surgery, with high rates in children under five, lowest in the 5–15 age range and then rising steadily with age to a second peak at about 70–74
- surgery contact rates for females were much higher than for males in the 16–64 age range
- rates for home visit contact for both doctors and nurses were extremely skewed towards patients over 70
- higher contact rates for men aged 16–64 in the north of England compared to the rest of the country; higher rates for people in the more deprived social classes IV and V compared to classes I and II; and higher rates for patients from the Indian subcontinent than white people.

The survey catalogued its own strengths and weaknesses. From the perspective of workload data, the key strengths were:

- a very large sample – 1% of England and Wales
- a wide geographical spread
- varied practices in terms of characteristics, though with the advantage of largely being experienced data recorders
- a full year's data and high reportage rates (96%) for doctor contacts
- direct linkage between each contact and its morbidity cause(s)
- combined with socio-economic data for 83% of patients.

The acknowledged weaknesses included:

- not a random sample of practices, relying instead on volunteers
- poor data recording by some practices for nurse contacts, with an average reportage of only 64%.

To this we would add:

- it is an expensive exercise and therefore is only done every ten years, which means the data becomes progressively out of date.

This is a serious issue at a time of rapid change in general practice

- it cannot detect local factors, for instance only one Sheffield practice participated
- since it is practices who choose to participate rather than patients, the self-selection could arguably lead to high-workload practices being under-represented because they could not face the extra demands of participating in the survey
- since it does not use data that is routinely generated by the everyday workings of the practice, it is hard for practices to use NMS data as a direct standard for benchmarking their own work.

The General Household Survey

The annual General Household Survey is a sample of about 25 000 individuals in 10 000 households in Great Britain which, amongst many other questions, asks them about their visits to the doctor over the last two weeks. Whilst this data set avoids the issue of GP bias by going direct to patients, there are problems in extrapolating from two weeks to 52 weeks. A greater concern is the reliability of peoples' memory recall over the two-week reference period. However, it has been shown to produce similar results to the National Morbidity Surveys.

The National Survey of NHS Patients

During October to December 1998 the first annual National Survey of NHS Patients in England was conducted. It was a self-completed questionnaire sent by post to a random sample of 100 000 adults from the electoral registers. Over 61 000 questionnaires were returned. The survey focused on patients' experience of general practice. Some of its questions were of relevance to studying consultation patterns – including details about contact with a GP or practice nurse, and waiting times to see a GP. As with the General Household Survey, it relies on peoples' memory recall. Reference to its findings are made at various points in this book.

Department of Health's General Practice Research Database (GPRD)

This routinely collects data from 288 practices who use the VAMP clinical computer system and have been deemed reliable and comprehensive in their clinical data collection. Whilst it is a potential source of information on GP activity, its use for research purposes has entirely focused on morbidity or pharmacology

A local approach?

In the last ten years, quite a number of projects have been set up to systematically collect data from many general practices in one area. Almost all of these projects have focused on the collection of morbidity data, and there now exists a national body that guides their work – the Collection of Health Data from General Practice (CHDGP) project. Rarely though has the focus been on workload. Our work in Sheffield has been an exception.

The Sheffield Practice Data Comparison (PDC) project

In 1989, eight geographically dispersed practices initiated the Towards Coordinated Practice (TCP) project, whose aim was to explore ways in which collaboration between practices could usefully assist the development of primary care. One of the ideas that emerged was the routine sharing and comparison of standardised practice-held data. The Practice Data Comparison project began in 1994 and was funded by Sheffield Health. Project workers were accountable to an independent management group and the project was clearly identified as of, and for, general practice. Data has been collected on activity rates, finances and morbidity, but the principal focus, decided by the general practices involved, has been on activity and workload issues. The results of the data comparison have been used to:

1   inform resource management decisions within practices
2   make accurate, anonymised data available to Sheffield Health about a broad patient base to inform the commissioning process
3   improve the appropriateness, accessibility, costs and quality of care given to patients.

Over time the project has expanded the number of participating practices so that we have at least one year's worth of data for 33 practices. The project is now a part of the Sheffield-based Centre for Innovation in Primary Care, which is a charity independent of NHS structures and commercial interests.

The initial reports presented the participating practices with comparative bar charts of annual data and commentaries, with the practices openly identified. These reports generated intra-practice discussion and sometimes were supplemented by multi-disciplinary meetings of all the practices where participants sought to understand the reasons for variation and learn from each other.

The next step was a series of reports entitled *Your Questions Answered*. Each of these short reports started from a practical question from somebody in a practice, e.g. 'how many days do our patients have to wait for an appointment?', and answered it within a comparative framework. A number of the chapters in this book grew out of such questions.

A further stage began in 1998, with funding from Trent National Health Service Executive (NHSE), to explore the potential of computer appointment systems as a routine source of activity data in combination with data from practice clinical databases about patients. This material forms the basis for a number of chapters in the second half of this book. The method of collecting this data is explained on page 65.

How representative is the data?

The Practice Data Comparison project has collected data on activity rates in 33 general practices that collectively serve 39% of Sheffield's population – nearly 200 000 patients. Although PDC practices are self-selected, this large sample is broadly representative of Sheffield practices in terms of deprivation, age structure, GP full-time equivalents/1000 patients and geographical spread. However, small practices are somewhat under-represented, as are practices on the western, less deprived edge of the city. In particular, there is only one single-handed practice in the project. It is likely that the data is probably representative of urban general practice in the UK in the late 1990s. It may be a less accurate reflection of practice in inner London and in rural areas. PDC now has a continuous data set for five years from four practices, and three years from 17 practices.

How reliable is the data?

The project was carefully designed to keep the workload in each practice to a minimum and certainly no more than two hours per month. A minimum data set that virtually all practices were already recording in some form was identified. Mostly this was being done by simply adding up weekly attendance and visiting figures for their own monitoring purposes. Practices were given a set of instructions and definitions (*see* Appendix 2 for the definitions). They were visited to discuss how to record the data in a standardised way and how, if necessary, their current recording systems should be modified or added to. A growing minority of practices are now able to provide the data on surgery consultations direct from their computer appointment or clinical system.

Paper-based counts of surgery consultations tend to include patients who failed to attend for their appointment but were not marked as a default (Did Not Attend, or DNA). However, they may tend to exclude consultations which were in the building but outside the normal schedule of surgeries and clinics. There was no pattern for practices with paper-based systems to have higher consultation rates than those with computer appointment systems. In the few cases where we were able to compare a paper record with a computer record for the same practice and time period, this suggested that the paper counts tended to be 3–5% higher.

Calculating consultation rates requires knowing the list size of the practice to act as the denominator in the calculation. We utilised practices' own data on list size. At first this was collected quarterly, more latterly annually as we found by experience that a quarterly snapshot made little difference to the final figure compared to an annual snapshot. It is well known that practices' own lists are inflated by 'ghost patients' who have left the area without informing the practice. Once they register with a new GP, which may not be for a while, the NHS system should detect the new registration and remove the patient from the practice list. This works more effectively if they move within the same health authority than if they move to another authority area. Patients who leave the country may be 'ghosts' for years.

Now that practices have a computer link to their health authority for the registering of patients, the scope for list inflation has been reduced. In recent years we have found that practice-supplied list sizes have averaged about 1% higher than figures supplied by the health authority. Inflation of lists, by increasing the denominator in the calculation, serves to slightly reduce the consultation rate.

Data on home visits is the least reliable. Visit books filled in by receptionists when patients request a visit may overestimate the number of acute visits if GPs fail to record where they phoned a patient back and never made a visit. They may be a poor record of visits initiated by the GP or nurse since this relies on the clinician making an entry. They may also be a poor record of out-of-hours visits since this also relies on the GP recording the visit later. In all it is safe to assume that our data on GP and practice nurse home visits is an underestimate of the actual visit rate. An initial distinction in our data collection between acute (patient-initiated) and non-acute or chronic (practice-initiated) visits was eventually abandoned because we felt that there were inconsistencies between practices in how they interpreted the distinction.

Records of visits by deputising services should be highly accurate since the service has a direct financial interest in accurate recording, and the practice has to do no more than transfer the data to our recording sheet.

The issue of the relationship between our results and those of the National Morbidity Survey is further discussed in Chapter 4.

Further information

Further information can be found in our reports:

- *Activity and Costs: collecting data on the hidden aspects of general practice*, September 1995
- *IT Could Be Better: implementing NSFs and HImPs with general practice IT systems*, October 1999.

Other useful reading

Fleming D (1989) Consultation rates in English general practice. *Journal of the Royal College of General Practitioners*. **39**: 68–72.

Over 10 years old but still the best overview of both the sources of data about general practice consultation rates, and their relative reliability.

Ebrahim S (1995) Changing patterns of consultation in general practice: Fourth National Morbidity Survey, 1991–1992, *British Journal of General Practice.* **45**: 283–5.
Summarises the key findings of the Morbidity Survey.

Aylin P, Majeed A and Cook D (1996) Home visiting by general practitioners in England and Wales. *BMJ.* **313**: 207–10.
Summarises the key findings of the Fourth National Morbidity Survey on home visits.

Howarth F, Maitland J and Duffus P (1989) Standardisation of core data for practice annual reports: a pilot study. *Journal of the Royal College of General Practitioners.* **39**: 463–6.
Outlines a potential comparative core data set for general practice. Our data set is a slimmed-down version of theirs.

Neal R, Heywood P and Morley S (1996) Real world data – retrieval and validation of consultation data from four general practices. *Family Practice.* **13**: 455–61.
Outlines the potential and difficulties of collecting activity data from general practice clinical databases using Miquest software.

Campbell S, Roland M and Gormanly B (1996) Evaluation of a computerised appointment system in general practice. *British Journal of General Practice.* **46**: 477–8.
Outlines the benefits of a computer appointment system for clinicians, receptionists and patients.

3 A day in the life of a typical urban general practice

What is it like working in a typical urban general practice? How many patients are seen, prescriptions issued, phone calls dealt with each day and week? Answering these questions is difficult because most of the necessary data is either not collected at all, or only on a local basis. This chapter provides a baseline understanding. Fuller details about many of the activity rates are presented in the chapters that follow. What follows is not a statistical average but a broad brush picture put together from a range of Sheffield and national data sources.

There are about 10 000 practices throughout the UK, varying in size from single-handed GPs with as few as 1000 patients through to group practices of more than ten doctors with perhaps as many as 25 000 patients. Data from the Department of Health's Statistics for General Medical Practitioners indicates that in 1998 the average English general practice had about four partners, and that the average list size for a full-time partner was 1979 patients. Therefore the average English practice had nearly 8000 patients. (In Scotland, Northern Ireland and Wales, individual list and practice sizes tend to be lower.)

Practices in large conurbations tend to be smaller. This means that in Sheffield in 1997 the average list size was 5428 patients. The tables that follow are, for simplicity, based on the Myrtle Road practice, an imaginary practice with 5000 patients and three full-time GPs. Activity rates are presented per year, per full working week, and per working weekday. The annual rate is also presented for 1000 patients since this is the way activity rates are conventionally presented in other publications.

Daytime contact rates

Table 3.1 shows that on a typical day at the Myrtle Road practice, 67 patients will be seen in the surgery building by a GP and 19 by a practice nurse. The GPs will make seven home visits during daytime working hours and the practice nurse one. In addition, four patients will default on their GP appointment (6%) and two on their nurse appointment (10%).

General practice workload varies with the time of year, though less than some might expect. The final figures in the weekday

Table 3.1: Myrtle Road daytime contact rates

	Per 1000 patients	Per 5000 patients		
	Annual	Annual	Working week	Weekday
GP surgery consultations	3385	16 925	337	67 (62–72)
Nurse surgery consultations	933	4665	93	19 (16–24)
GP weekday daytime home visits	352	1760	35	7 (6–9)
Nurse daytime home visits	36	180	4	1
GP defaulted appointments (DNAs)	208	1040	21	4
Nurse defaulted appointments (DNAs)	101	505	10	2

All figures rounded to the nearest whole number. The working week figures allow for bank holidays. The weekday figures allow for a small amount of GP activity on a Saturday.

The figures on consultations and visits are based on aggregate data from 29 Sheffield practices, April 1997–March 1998. The figures on DNAs are based on detailed computer appointment data from nine Sheffield practices for 1997.

column show how the contact rates may vary according to seasonal highs and lows. For instance, in January the GPs may have 72 consultations per day and nine home visits whilst in August it falls to 62 consultations and six visits. Actual daily contact rates vary quite a lot around the average. The only predictable pattern to this is that Mondays are the highest workload day, after the weekend surgery closure. Typically, 25% of the week's GP consultations and home visits occur on a Monday.

Out-of-hours contact rates

How requests for evening, night-time, weekend and bank holiday visits are dealt with varies. Increasingly, though, most or all of this service is provided by a deputising service which may be a GP cooperative or a commercial company. In Sheffield it is now principally provided by a GP co-op. Table 3.2 shows the out-of-hours demand at our imaginary Myrtle Road.

Table 3.2: **Myrtle Road out-of-hours contacts with GP co-op**			
	Per 1000 patients	Per 5000 patients	
	Annual	Annual	Working week
Night visits	9	45	1
Night surgery consultations	10	50	1
Day visits	24	110	2
Day surgery consultations	46	230	4
Advice calls	93	465	9

All figures rounded to the nearest whole number. The working week figures allow for bank holidays.
The figures are based on aggregate data from 23 Sheffield practices, April 1998–March 1999.

During an average week the co-op will receive 17 calls from Myrtle Road patients, of which nine will be dealt with by advice only, five will result in the patient visiting the co-op's own surgery and only three will require a visit.

Receptionist activity rates

Perhaps the busiest people in a surgery are the receptionists. We know of no organisation that has systematically collected data on receptionist workload across practices, but data from two Sheffield practices allows us to present a rough picture of the scale of their activity (Table 3.3).

During an average day the Myrtle Road receptionists will deal with 158 incoming telephone calls, file 57 letters or lab tests in patient notes and process 34 requests for repeat prescriptions. They will spend 3 hours 25 minutes dealing with the incoming calls (an average of 1 minute 18 seconds per call). They will handle a Lloyd George patient record twice for each surgery appointment and home visit (getting out and putting back), once for each letter filed, twice for some of the repeat scripts processed, and a few records for other reasons. This involves pulling or filing a set of notes about 300 times per day. Each surgery consultation will involve one and sometimes two face-to-face contacts (for booking a future appointment), as will each repeat prescription, and there will be some other contacts, e.g. registering patients. This amounts to around 160 face-to-face contacts per day.

Some of this workload has implications for GPs. One GP will have dealt with the 34 repeat prescriptions, whilst at least one and maybe all of the GPs will have read the 57 letters and lab tests.

Table 3.3:   Myrtle Road receptionist activity rates

	Per 1000 patients	Per 5000 patients		
	Annual	Annual	Working week	Weekday
(a) Incoming telephone calls	8126	40 630	809	158
(b) Patient letters and lab tests filed	2890	14 450	288	57
(c) Repeat scripts processed	1750	8750	174	34
(d) Patient records processed	15 360	76 800	1530	300
(e) Reception face-to-face contacts	8200	41 000	817	160

All figures rounded to the nearest whole number. The working week figures allow for bank holidays. The weekday figures allow for a small amount of GP activity on a Saturday.
Row (a) is based on a telephone meter survey by one Sheffield practice for five months in 1999.
Rows (b) and (c) are based on annual data from another Sheffield practice for 1998.
Rows (d) and (e) are estimates from other data – *see* page 18.

Other rates

Each of the 34 repeat prescriptions issued will contain anything from one to maybe ten items. Add in the acute prescriptions issued during consultations and you have in excess of 200 items pre-scribed and then actually obtained from a pharmacist during the working day. (The English as opposed to Sheffield average would be about 175.) The number of referrals to hospitals is three per day, though this omits letters/referrals to community trusts and other agencies. This means that about one in every 23 GP consultations (4.4%) resulted in a hospital referral.

Table 3.4 indicates that in an average week 21 of Myrtle Road's patients will be admitted to hospital by all the possible routes, one will die, one baby will be born, and including the birth and death about nine people will leave the list and another nine join. It also indicates that 23% of Myrtle Road's patients will not see a GP or practice nurse during the year. This will particularly be the case for young men who as a group have the lowest consultation rates. By contrast, 65 patients (1.3% of the list) will attend the surgery 20 or

Table 3.4:   Other Myrtle Road rates

	Per 1000 patients	Per 5000 patients		
	Annual	Annual	Working week	Weekday
Items prescribed	10 700	53 500	1066	209
Hospital referrals	150	750	15	3
Hospital admissions	216	1080	21	–
Deaths	12	60	1	–
Live births	11	55	1	–
Patients leaving and joining the list	90 patients	450	9	–
Non-attenders	230 patients	1150	–	–
20 or more attendances	13 patients	65	–	–

All figures rounded to the nearest whole number. The working week figures allow for bank holidays. The weekday figures allow for a small amount of GP activity on a Saturday.

Data on attendance comes from comprehensive computer appointment data for nine Sheffield practices in 1998. Items prescribed is based on the Sheffield average for April 1998 to March 1999 – from Prescription Pricing Authority data. The other data is from Sheffield Health and is the Sheffield average for April 1996 to March 1997.

more times, in the process generating 8.3% of the practice's workload.

Practice staffing

With 5000 urban patients, Myrtle Road will probably be classified as having three full-time equivalent partners. This will still probably be three full-time GPs. However, part-time working is steadily increasing amongst GPs, up from 5% in 1990 to 16% in 1998. Also growing steadily is the percentage of GPs who are female, up from 22% in 1988 to 31% in 1998. We can reasonably assume that one of Myrtle Road's GPs is a woman.

Based on national averages for 1998, Myrtle Road will have 38 hours of practice nursing – probably two part-time nurses rather than one full-timer – and 180 hours of administrative staff time – receptionists, secretary, practice manager, computer operator, etc. (Table 3.5). This amounts in total to the equivalent of two full-time staff per full-time GP. This represents a major expansion from 1988 when the practice would have had only 13 nursing and 110 administrative hours – little more than one full-time equivalent per GP. The bulk of this expansion, especially in nursing hours, occurred in 1988–1993, and has slowed since.

Table 3.5: Myrtle Road staffing		
	Per 1000 patients	Per 5000 patients
Practice nurse hours	7.6	38
Admin and reception hours	36	180

Data for 1998 derived from the Department of Health statistical bulletin – *Statistics for General Medical Practitioners in England: 1988–1998.*

4 Are GP surgery consultation rates rising?

GPs regularly complain about rising workload. Many assume therefore that in recent years they have been seeing more patients. Is this true? In Sheffield at least the answer is no. Table 4.1 shows the aggregate GP surgery consultation rate per 1000 patients for 17 practices for three consecutive calendar years, and for four practices for five years going back to 1994. For these practices rates vary between static and showing a small drop. It should also be noted, though, that the rates are over 30% higher than the figure of 2622 recorded in the 1991/2 National Morbidity Survey.

Figure 4.1 presents recent data for 27 practices. It shows the range of consultation rates – from 2482 to 3990 per 1000 patients. For 23 of the practices it also compares their rate during the period April 1st 1998–March 31st 1999 (the column) with their rate during the previous year (the horizontal bar). Seventeen practices registered a (generally) small decline in consultation rate whilst only six showed a small increase.

Our data set covers the second half of the 1990s but for two practices we can look back further. One Sheffield practice participated in the 1991/2 NMS which recorded every surgery consultation. Since 1996 it has used a computer appointment system to log every consultation. We were therefore able to compare its GP consultation rate in the late 1990s with its rate in 1991/2, using exactly the same method of calculation. The rates were virtually identical – there had been no increase. A second practice has kept its own paper record of consultations since 1979. Its rate in 1996 was also virtually identical to its rate in 1990.

Table 4.1: Annual GP surgery consultation rate per 1000 patients

Year	17 practices	4 practices
1994	–	3635
1995	–	3631
1996	3462	3662
1997	3387	3639
1998	3364	3519

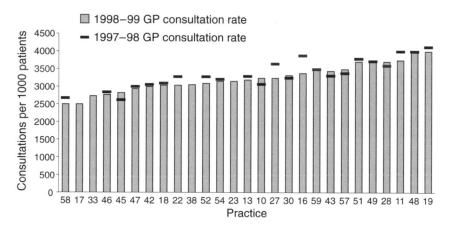

Figure 4.1: Annual GP surgery consultation rate, April 1st 1997–March 31st 1999.

If GP consultation rates are not rising, why are the Sheffield rates much higher than the national survey?

The average consultation rates that we have recorded have consistently been 30% or more higher than those found in the 1991/2 National Morbidity Survey. If consultation rates have not risen since 1991, what might account for these differences? We have identified three broad reasons.

Different counting methods?

The PDC definition of a 'consultation' was identical to the NMS definition of a 'contact'. The NMS used the word consultation to refer to the reason for the contact. Since some contacts had more than one reason, a single contact might be two or even three consultations. The average was 1.2 consultations per contact.

The NMS estimated that it only captured 96% of GP surgery contacts and therefore *underestimated* true consultation rates by 4%. It also omitted the small number of consultations by temporary residents. A validation of our paper-based data collection methods in four practices with computer appointment systems suggested that the PDC data was a 3% *overestimate.*

Different practice populations?

The two surveys had largely similar populations in terms of age and sex, and recalculating the results to allow for the small differences had negligible effect on the difference in consultation rates. However, various studies have shown that on average poorer people consult more than wealthier people. Sheffield, as a big city, is more deprived than the England and Wales average. There is no simple formula for calculating how much in excess of the national average one would expect Sheffield's consultation rates to be. However, it is reasonable to assume that a significant part of the 30% extra consultations in Sheffield can be accounted for by the city's higher levels of socio-economic deprivation.

Different kinds of practice?

Both surveys were based on volunteer practices and under-represented smaller, and particularly single-handed, practices. Participation in the PDC data collection demanded very little from practices, many of whom were collecting much of the information anyway. The NMS, however, involved a significant amount of extra work since data had to be logged for every contact and clinical problem encountered by the practice for a whole year. Whilst the practices received some extra resources for the survey, this arguably did not fully compensate them for the work. This may create a bias in the NMS against high workload practices volunteering.

Further information

Further information can be found in our report:

* *Practice Consultation and Contact Rates: are they changing?* December 1999.

Key points

* The broad picture in Sheffield is one of static GP consultation rates during the 1990s, with some suggestion of a small decline towards the end of the decade. The evidence for an increase is non-existent.
* The average rates are, however, about 30% higher than those recorded in the 1991/2 National Morbidity Survey. This is probably due to the higher levels of deprivation in Sheffield, some difference in counting method and possibly to the NMS under-representing high workload practices.

What others have found

Allan K, Murphy P and Edwards R (1995) *Medics Scheme Practice Feedback Report.* Northumberland Health Authority, March 1995.
The average GP surgery consultation rate amongst 33 rural practices in Northumberland in 1994 was 3302 per 1000 patients.

5 If consultation rates are static, why do GPs complain about rising workload?

GPs think that they are having to work under increasing pressure. We actually agree – but to be able to respond effectively to the pressure, GPs need to understand its real origins.

From the beginning, the PDC project has sought to use comparative data to enable practitioners to better understand their situation, and learn from each other. As well as producing reports, we have organised occasional multi-disciplinary meetings of participating practices to discuss those reports. The title question for this chapter was put to two meetings in Sheffield in April 1998, involving in total 15 GPs, seven practice managers and one practice nurse. Participants had seen the data showing static GP surgery consultation rates. First of all they were asked whether they believed the data, and they did. The discussion that followed explored the seeming paradox of static consultation rates but a perceived rising workload. Three broad explanations were identified.

1 The GPs present suggested that demand was rising but rather than providing more consultations they were finding other ways to meet it. These **coping strategies** included:

- recalling patients less frequently for checks. The response to an acute illness was no longer 'come back in a week and we'll see how you are' but rather 'if it has not cleared up within a week, make another appointment'
- dealing with more problems by telephone
- delegating work to other health professionals, particularly practice nurses
- lengthening the review periods for repeat medication.

Some of these strategies may be very sensible, but the risk of coping responses is that corners get cut and risks taken.

Since most practice consultations are now arranged by advance appointment, the number of appointments offered was seen as putting a crude cap on the number of consultations. Whilst busy GP surgeries are experienced as being demand-led, in reality practices are taking broad decisions about how many consultations they are prepared to supply.

2 **Paperwork** was universally seen as having increased dramatically in the 1990s. For example:

- a major increase in repeat prescriptions issued
- a similar major increase in correspondence from hospital and community trusts
- the demands of the 1990 GP contract
- more demand from other agencies, e.g. letters for the housing department, insurance forms, sick notes for employee absence after only two days, benefits agency forms, etc.

Data is presented in Figure 5.1 to show how, for one Sheffield practice, the number of repeat prescriptions issued and the number of incoming hospital letters and lab tests per patient roughly doubled over the period 1989–1994, though it levelled off after that.

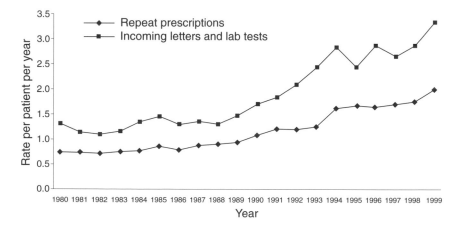

Figure 5.1: A Sheffield practice's paperwork.

Participants commented that the introduction of computer transfer of much paperwork between practices and the health authority had not meant any reduction in the work involved at the practice end in processing registration and item-of-service data.

3 It was agreed that the **complexity of consultations** had increased. This was felt to be due to:

- patients having higher expectations and wanting more detailed explanations
- hospitals appeared to have adopted some of the same coping strategies as GPs, for instance they were doing less routine follow-up and instead expected GPs to do it
- as hospital departments become more specialised it was felt that GPs are *de facto* replacing the hospital-based general physician. Consequently they are having more consultations that deal with multi-system problems
- the shift of work to practice nurses was occurring for the simpler illnesses or for well-controlled chronic conditions, leaving GPs' work more concentrated at the complex end of the spectrum
- some GPs felt that consultations over 'unnecessary' sick notes or housing letters were stressful because it put them in a double bind. They did not believe they should be undertaking the consultation, but recognised that if they did not the patient would suffer.

In short, the decision density in practice consultations is likely to be rising.

Much of this shift in responsibilities may be entirely appropriate when viewing the NHS as a whole. Experienced GPs perhaps should be the general physicians of the future. The sense of resentment in the meetings came from the feeling that this change was happening in an unplanned way, without acknowledgement and without a transfer of resources.

Further information

Further information can be found in our report:

- *Learning from comparative data: a report of two meetings*, June 1998.

Key points

- GPs attributed their perceived rise in workload to a mixture of increased paperwork and increased complexity of consultations.
- They felt that the demand for consultations was rising but that they were adopting various coping strategies to meet the demand in other ways, e.g. telephone consultations, nurse consultations, undertaking fewer check-ups.

What others have found

Pedersen LL and Leese B (1997) What will a primary care-led NHS mean for GP workload? The problem of the lack of an evidence base. *BMJ.* **314:** 1337–41.

A literature review found little hard evidence that the shift from secondary to primary care had increased GP workload.

Leese B, Pedersen LL and Holden J (1997) Burden of proof. *Health Services Journal.* **27 Nov:** 34–5.

Explored the use of a diary method with one GP to measure in detail the changes in GP workload due to the transfer of activity from secondary care.

Scott A and Vale L (1998) Increased general practice workload due to a primary care-led National Health Service: the need for evidence to support rhetoric. *British Journal of General Practice.* **48:** 1085–8.

A literature review on the shifting of work from secondary to primary care concluded that the effect on activity rates had been negligible, but the studies may have failed to capture other qualitative and quantitative changes in work.

Scott A and Wordsworth S (1999) The effects of shifts in the balance of care on general practice workload. *Family Practice.* **16:** 12–17.

The view of 52 Grampian GPs surveyed was that their workload was increasing due to changes in the balance of care. This was primarily due to geriatric and nursing home care, early discharge from hospital and changes in psychiatric and psychology services. They had responded by shifting tasks onto practice nurses and absorbing the workload into existing practices/patterns.

Bain J (1998) Relationship between new and return consultations and workload in general practice. *British Journal of General Practice.* **48:** 1855.

GPs in Tayside with higher surgery workloads tended to have a greater proportion of return consultations. They could perhaps reduce their workload by recalling fewer patients.

Telephone consultations

Brown A and Armstrong D (1995) Telephone consultations in general practice: an additional or alternative service. *British Journal of General Practice.* **45:** 673–5.

Sixty-three per cent of patient users of a practice phone-in clinic felt their telephone consultation substituted for a surgery consultation (53%) or a home visit (10%), whilst 5% felt it was an additional service and 32% were unsure.

Hallam L (1993) Access to general practice and general practitioners by telephone: the patient's view. *British Journal of General Practice.* **43:** 331–5.

Satisfaction with the help received from GPs by telephone was high in all four practices surveyed. However, many patients were unaware that they could have a telephone consultation, and over half reported being unable to get through to the surgery on their first attempt. A standard of one incoming line per 2500 patients was recommended.

Nagle J, McMahon K, Barbour M *et al.* (1991) Evaluation of the use and usefulness of telephone consultations in one general practice. *British Journal of General Practice.* **42:** 190–3.

Seventy-five per cent of the calls to the advice line of one practice would have otherwise required a surgery consultation and 13% would have required a home visit.

Stuart A, Rogers S and Modell M (2000) Evaluation of a direct doctor–patient telephone advice line in general practice. *British Journal of General Practice.* **50:** 305–6.

A GP-staffed direct access telephone line for 30 minutes each morning in one practice was valued by patients, but the reduction in surgery consultations achieved was not worth the input of GP time.

Box 5.1: Taking a longer view

It is clear that over the last 40 years or so the profession has given away, or is in the process of giving away, large parts of what GPs traditionally did:

- obstetric and antenatal care is now largely in the hands of hospitals and midwives
- palliative care is now often carried out by Macmillan nurses and hospices
- out-of-hours work is delivered by co-ops and deputising services
- minor illness is increasingly triaged by nurses and NHS Direct
- care of chronic illness is falling under the care of systematic review carried out by practice nurses
- practice-based counselling services are more available than they used to be.

In their place has come:

- more mental illness – the closure of large institutions means that more people with serious mental illness are now looked after in the community

- much more powerful therapeutics
- more geriatric care within nursing and residential homes
- more complex consultations – an older population with more co-morbidity, higher expectations, more therapeutic options and high rates of technical and organisational change
- resource management roles – fundholding may have been replaced by work for PCGs, but the pressure to use resources to best advantage remains
- increased accountability – clinical governance and the Commission for Health Improvement
- increased consistency – Health Improvement Programmes (HImPs) and National Service Frameworks (NSFs)
- breaking up of the single General Medical Services (GMS) based contract.

And in the future, primary care will be called on to deal with ever more powerful therapeutics, pharmacogenomics, much more near patient testing, genetic screening and more effective screening for many major diseases.

All this means that GPs are under severe role strain. The old ways of perceiving and valuing GP work no longer fit, whilst the new feel temporary and frequently contradict the older models.

6 What is happening to practice nurse consultation rates?

During the late 1980s and the early 1990s there was a major expansion in the employment of practice nurses. The number of whole-time equivalent practice nurses in England grew from 3480 in 1988 to 9605 in 1993. In the second half of the decade the numbers have continued to grow but at a much slower rate, reaching 10 358 in 1998 (data from *Statistics for General Medical Practitioners*, Department of Health). What has this meant for consultation rates with practice nurses?

Table 6.1 shows the aggregate practice nurse surgery consultation rate per 1000 patients for 17 Sheffield practices for three consecutive calendar years, and for four practices for five years going back to 1994. For these practices the evidence is of rates that are broadly static.

Figure 6.1 presents data for 28 practices. It shows a more than threefold variation in consultation rates – from 457 to 1549 per 1000 patients. It also compares for 24 of the practices their rate during the period April 1st 1998–March 31st 1999 (the column) with their rate during the previous year (the horizontal bar). Sixteen practices registered a decline in consultation rate, whilst eight showed an increase.

The inter-practice variation in practice nurse consultation rates is much greater than for GPs (compare Figure 6.1 with Figure 4.1). The year-to-year changes in rate within an individual practice also tend to be greater.

Whilst GPs can exert some control over their workload by the number of surgeries provided and appointments offered, they are

Table 6.1: Annual practice nurse surgery consultation rate per 1000 patients

Year	17 practices	4 practices
1994	–	866
1995	–	779
1996	883	881
1997	927	924
1998	908	908

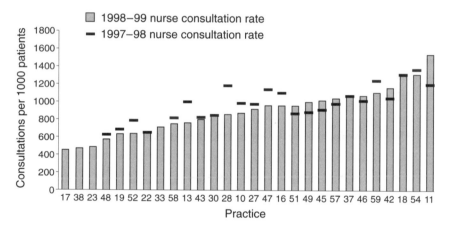

Figure 6.1: Annual practice nurse surgery consultation rate, April 1st 1997–March 31st 1999.

also responding to patient demand. The desire to see a GP remains the core pressure on general practice in Britain. Thus GP consultation rates are the result of a complex interaction between demand and supply.

With practice nursing the situation is different. It is, relatively speaking, a new service and GPs, as the employer, take decisions about how many hours of practice nursing to provide. There is a wide variation in that provision. Amongst the Sheffield PDC practices in 1998, the number of nursing hours per 1000 patients ranged from 5.3 to 12.4. Seventy-four per cent of the variation in practice nurse consultation rates in Sheffield can be explained by the variation in the supply of nursing hours. Further, the rates bear no relation at all to factors affecting the populations the practices serve, such as age structure or level of deprivation.

Our data set covers the second half of the 1990s and once again shows no evidence for an increase in consultation rates. However, the main growth in practice nursing occurred during the late 1980s and early 1990s. The Sheffield practice that participated in the 1991/2 National Morbidity Survey registered a 100% increase in its practice nurse consultation rate between 1991 and 1997 (even after allowing for the under-recording by the NMS). For the practice that has kept its own paper record of consultations since 1979, its practice nurse consultation rate barely changed during the early 1990s. However, its rate had already jumped by 150% during the second half of the 1980s. In both cases the dramatic increase coincided with the expansion of the number of nursing hours employed in the practice.

To explore this issue further, we analysed comprehensive computer appointment data from nine Sheffield practices for approximately 46 000 consultations in-surgery with a practice nurse during 1998. Their average consultation rate with a practice nurse in-surgery was close to the PDC average. This was compared with data from the 1991/2 National Morbidity Survey.

The raw age-specific nurse consultation rates from the NMS were adjusted upwards to allow for the 36% of consultations that the NMS missed. They were then applied to the patient base of the Sheffield study practices to calculate what the number of consultations *would have been* in nine practices with the same age structure in 1991. These hypothesised figures for 1991 were then compared with the actual age-specific consultation rates in the Sheffield practices in 1998. Overall, the figures for Sheffield in 1998 were 86% higher.

Table 6.2 presents the percentage difference by age group. Whilst the Sheffield figures are higher across the entire age range, this was

Table 6.2: Percentage difference in nurse consultations, 1991 to 1998

Age group	0–4	5–15	16–24	25–44	45–64	65–74	75–84	85+	Total
% extra 1998	36%	91%	120%	91%	82%	91%	86%	124%	86%

Table 6.3: Comparison of nursing employment

	Weekly nursing hours per 1000 patients	Nurse consultations per hour of work
NMS practices 1991	7.0	1.56
Sheffield study practices 1998	9.3	2.20

The final column of Table 6.3 assumes 45 weeks a year actually working (with no replacement), the rest taken as holidays and bank holidays.

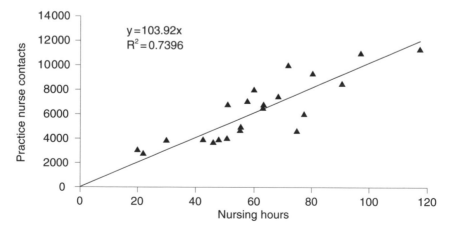

Figure 6.2: Practice nurse contacts vs. nursing hours.

least amongst the under-fives and greatest in the 16–24 and 85+ age ranges.

Is this higher level in Sheffield simply a function of more nurses employed? Table 6.3 presents comparative data from the two surveys on both the numbers of nursing hours and the number of consultations undertaken per hour.

Table 6.3 shows that the 86% more consultations in the Sheffield study can be attributed to the combined effect of 33% more nurses employed and 41% more patients seen per hour compared to the NMS practices. The reason(s) for the higher throughput of patients cannot be definitively identified but may be partly due to nurses doing more very short consultations to vaccinate patients against influenza compared to 1991.

Figure 6.2 further explores the issue of how many patients practice nurses see per hour of work. It plots the relationship between the number of nursing hours in each practice in 1997 and the number of face-to-face contacts, in surgery or at home, between a patient and a practice nurse during the year April 1st 1996–March 31st 1997. Home visits were counted as a double contact in recognition of the extra time they take, though they accounted for only 4% of the total number of contacts.

The sloping line on Figure 6.2 (in statistical terminology, the regression line) plots the average number of yearly contacts for each nursing hour – about 104 yearly contacts per hour of nursing employment (on average 96 surgery consultations and four 'double contact' home visits). It represents the statistical 'best fit' with the data, subject to the constraint that it should logically pass through the 0,0 point on the chart since practices with no nurses will have no nurse contacts. Practices above the line have a higher contact rate per annual hour of nurse employment than the average, those below the line a lower contact rate. The R^2 value indicates that about 74% of the variation between practices in the number of nurse contacts can be statistically accounted for by the number of nursing hours.

A narrow 'time and motion' interpretation of this chart would conclude that practices with high contact rates per hour are using their nursing hours more 'efficiently'. However, low contact rates may be the result of clear policy decisions, such as to have longer nurse consultation times, to run patient groups or to have nurses taking on a greater number of administrative tasks. In the absence of health outcome measures, no judgement can be made about the appropriateness of any approach.

Further information

Further information can be found in our reports:

- *Practice Consultation and Contact Rates: are they changing?* December 1999.
- *What Do Practice Nurses Do?* September 2000.
- *How Does Our Nursing Administrative Staff Provision Compare With Other Practices in PDC?* November 1997.

Key points

- Practice nurse consultation rates are principally a function of the number of nursing hours employed.
- Nationally, the big increase in practice nurse hours occurred in the period 1988–1993.
- Practice nurse consultation rates in Sheffield have been largely static in the second half of the 1990s.
- There is evidence that there has been a major increase in practice nurse consultation rates since 1991. This is likely to have occurred in the first half of the decade.
- There is also evidence that the number of nurse consultations per hour worked has increased significantly since 1991.

What others have found

Hirst M, Lunt N and Atkin K (1998) Were practice nurses distributed equitably across England and Wales, 1988–1995? *Journal of Health Services Research Policy.* **3**: 31–8.

There was a twofold variation in nurse numbers per 1000 patients at the health authority level which could not be attributed to a variation in health needs.

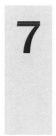

7 What is happening to GP home visits?

National evidence indicates that GP daytime home visiting has been in decline for several decades. What has been happening recently in Sheffield?

Table 7.1 shows the aggregate GP 'daytime' home visit rate per 1000 patients for 17 Sheffield practices for three consecutive calendar years, and for four practices for five years going back to 1994. This includes all visits undertaken by a GP except those between 10 p.m. and 8 a.m. which are classified as night visits. It also excludes visits undertaken during daytime hours by a deputising service. The data therefore principally represents the home visiting workload of GPs during their Monday to Friday, and Saturday morning, daytime working week, with some addition for the comparatively small number of on-call visits in the evening and at weekends. Our data indicates that in 1995 approximately three-quarters of these visits were 'acute visits' in response to a request by the patient on that day. The remainder were practice-initiated and will principally be visits to elderly patients with chronic illness.

For these practices the evidence is of rates that have been steadily declining.

We fed back this data to a discussion group of some of the participating GPs. They identified the following reasons for the decline in home visiting:

- as a conscious coping strategy they were initiating fewer visits, for instance by doing less visiting of the elderly with chronic illness

Table 7.1: Annual GP 'daytime' home visit rate per 1000 patients

Year	17 practices	4 practices
1994	–	720 (730)
1995	–	650 (662)
1996	420 (445)	576 (585)
1997	375 (421)	525 (574)
1998	344 (392)	463 (515)

Rates in brackets include all daytime visits by a commercial deputising service or GP co-op plus daytime consultations at the co-op's own surgery.

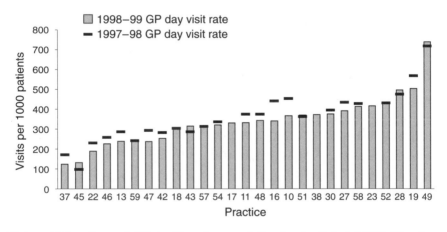

Figure 7.1: Annual GP daytime home visit rate, April 1st 1997–March 31st 1999.

- they were also more inclined to telephone patients who had requested a daytime home visit to see whether the visit was really necessary
- the introduction of the Sheffield GP cooperative for out-of-hours work in October 1996 had changed patients' expectations towards home visiting. The greater emphasis the co-op had placed on accepting telephone advice or coming to their night

surgery had rubbed off on patients' expectations during the daytime as well

- GPs were also now leaving more weekend and evening on-call cover to the co-op than they had done when the alternative was a commercial deputising service.

The figures in brackets in Table 7.1 indicate that taking allowance of the increase in daytime home visits by the GP co-op reduces the level of decline in daytime home visits but doesn't alter the fundamental trend.

Figure 7.1 presents recent data for 27 practices. It shows the range of home visit rates – from 126 to 746 per 1000 patients. It also compares for 23 of the practices their rate during the period April 1st 1998–March 31st 1999 (the column) with their rate during the previous year (the horizontal bar). Seventeen practices registered a generally small decline in visit rates whilst only seven showed a small increase.

It should be noted that even after a number of years of decline the rates in Sheffield are still significantly higher than the figure of 299 recorded in the 1991/2 NMS for *all* types of doctor home visit, including night visits and daytime visits by a deputising service.

Analysis of the two practices with data from 1991 showed that the practice which participated in the NMS had a similar GP visit rate in 1996 as in 1991, whilst the other practice's daytime home-visit rates had been largely static during the 1985–94 period, with a decline setting in after 1994.

Exploring daytime home visits in greater depth

In October 1996 we undertook an in-depth survey of *all* requests for home visits in eight practices for two weeks (Table 7.2). As expected, this showed that a large percentage of out-of-hours requests for home visits were dealt with by telephone advice

Table 7.2: What happened to visit requests		
	In-surgery hours	Out-of-hours
Not visited	42 (8%)	89 (47%)
Visited but inappropriate	131 (26%)	32 (17%)
Visited and appropriate	335 (66%)	69 (36%)

alone (47%). However, this was only true for 8% of daytime requests. Of the remaining 92%, the visiting GP deemed after the event that 66% were appropriate requests and 26% had not in their opinion needed a visit. Whilst most visit requests were from the elderly, the likelihood of a visit being deemed 'inappropriate' was much higher amongst visits to children (62%) than for the adult and elderly population.

During daytime hours it was rare that a telephone request for a visit was put directly through to a GP and most GPs made no attempt to telephone the patient back before visiting. They accepted that if the receptionist had taken the request then the patient needed visiting.

However, in two of the practices the GPs had adopted a strategy of telephoning back some of the patients before visiting. Forty-four per cent of the patients were rung back, and of these about half were not subsequently visited. Doubtless the GPs concerned exercised some degree of selection over who they rang back. There will be, for instance, patients whose history is known, patients whose symptoms clearly indicate a visit, and patients who do not have a telephone. However, this small survey indicated that perhaps a quarter of requests for daytime home visits could be dealt with by telephone advice alone.

Daytime visit requests were not evenly spread during the day and week. Twenty-eight per cent of the Monday to Friday requests came on the Monday, with the other four days ranging from 16–19%. As expected, the requests were heavily concentrated in the morning: 9–10 a.m. was the peak time with 35% of visit requests logged. Extending outwards from this, 57% of requests were between 8.30 and 10.30 a.m., and 67% between 8 and 11 a.m.

Further information

Further information can be found in our reports:

* *Practice Consultation and Contact Rates: are they changing?* December 1999.
* *Could I Have a Visit?* May 1997.

Key points

* GP daytime home visiting rates in Sheffield have been in steady decline in the late 1990s.
* However, they remain markedly higher than the national rate in the 1991/2 National Morbidity Survey.
* There is evidence to suggest that perhaps a quarter of daytime home visit requests could be dealt with by telephone advice.

What others have found

Aylin P, Majeed A and Cook D (1996) Home visiting by general practitioners in England and Wales. *BMJ.* 1996, **313**: 207–10.
Compared home-visit rates from the 1991 and 1981 National Morbidity Surveys. Found a 27% drop from 411 per 1000 patients to 299. In 1991, individual practice rates varied from 84 to 654.

Beale N (1991) Daily home visiting in one general practice: a longitudinal study of patient-initiated workload. *British Journal of General Practice.* **41**: 16–18.
Found a steady decline in patient-initiated demand for home visits

from 1977 to 1989 in one rural practice – from 219 per 1000 to 139. However, the decline was entirely in the 0–64 age range. Demand from patients over 65 had not decreased.

Jones K, Gilbert P, Little J *et al.* (1998) Nurse triage for house call requests in a Tyneside general practice: patients; views and effect on doctor workload. *British Journal of General Practice.* **48**: 1303–6.

Over 15 months, practice nurses triaged all daytime home visit requests. Only 41% ultimately required a home visit, 18% came to a GP surgery consultation and the rest were dealt with by nurse or GP telephone advice. Eighty per cent of patients reported satisfaction with the help received from the nurse.

8 What difference does a GP cooperative make to night visits?

Whilst daytime home visits had been in steady decline nationally, there was lots of evidence in the 1980s and early 1990s that night visits, whilst much fewer by comparison, were steadily increasing. The second half of the 1990s saw the widespread introduction of GP cooperatives to undertake night and other out-of-hours cover. These co-ops typically offer patients a mixture of telephone advice, home visits and consultations at the co-op's own surgery. What effect has this had on how night and other out-of hours visit requests are dealt with?

The Sheffield GP out-of-hours cooperative began in November 1996 and most Sheffield practices joined it, whilst some continued to undertake their own cover or to use a commercial deputising service. Previously, night cover had been a mixture of direct GP provision and use of the commercial deputising service. Many practices also handed over much of their non-night out-of-hours cover to the co-op.

Table 8.1 shows the effect on night visits for 13 practices for which we have data spanning the period before and after the beginning of the co-op. The 1996 rate of 41.9 night visits per 1000 patients is broadly comparable with other studies at the time. The data shows a substantial 74% drop in home visits after the introduction of the co-op. Only about one-third of this drop can be accounted for by the use of the option of attending a night surgery. It seems reasonable to assume that this drop in home visiting is due to many more night calls being dealt with by telephone advice than when the calls were handled by GPs or the

Table 8.1:   Annual night visit rates per 1000 patients

	Night home visits	Night surgery contacts	Total night contacts
1996	41.9	0.4	42.3
1997	18.7	8.9	27.6
1998	10.4	10.1	20.5

commercial deputising service. Unfortunately, we lack comparable data on the number of night calls that were and are dealt with by telephone advice only.

The Sheffield GP co-op also provides 'daytime' out-of-hours cover, such as during the evening, at weekends and bank holidays. Table 8.2 shows how the co-op responded to *all* visit requests for the same 13 practices. The overall number of requests fell slightly by 3% between 1997 and 1998 – from 181.9 calls per 1000 patients to 176.5. However, the percentage that resulted in a home visit fell markedly, with more calls leading to a consultation in the surgery at the co-op centre or being dealt with by advice only. The overall breakdown of responses is similar to that found in a much larger study by Salisbury *et al.* (2000).

Figure 8.1 presents recent data for 23 practices. It shows the range of night visit rates – from seven to 46 per 1000 patients.

Table 8.2:   GP co-op response to all visit requests

	Home visit	Surgery consultation	Advice only
11 Sheffield practices 1997	25.0%	24.6%	50.4%
11 Sheffield practices 1998	18.1%	29.0%	52.9%
20 co-op study 1997–98	23.6%	29.8%	45.4%

Final row data from a study of 20 English and Scottish GP co-ops – September 1997 to August 1998.

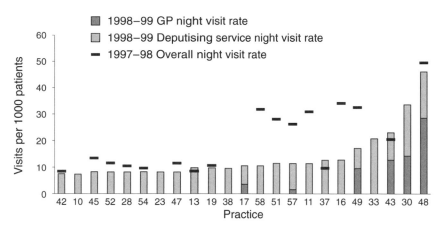

Figure 8.1: Annual night visit rate, April 1st 1998–March 31st 1999.

Interestingly, of the five practices with the highest night visit rates, four continue to undertake about half their own night visits. It also compares the rate for the 17 practices during the period April 1st 1998–March 31st 1999 (the column) with their rate during the previous year (the horizontal bar). Fourteen practices registered a decline in night visit rates whilst only three showed a small increase. The data indicates that the decline in night visits is continuing rather than being a one-off drop when the system changed.

Note

All our figures predate the introduction of NHS Direct into Sheffield. Evidence from the early sites suggests that it may be making a tiny reduction in the demand on GP out-of-hours cooperatives. *See*:

Munro J, Nicholl J, O'Cathain A *et al.* (2000) Impact of NHS Direct on demand for immediate care: observational study. *BMJ.* **321**: 150–3.

Further information

Further information can be found in our report:

* *Practice Consultation and Contact Rates: are they changing?* December 1999.

Key points

• The introduction in Sheffield of a GP out-of-hours cooperative has lead to a dramatic 74% drop in the number of night visits to patient homes. Only a third of this drop can be accounted for by an increase in the number of patients attending the co-op's night surgery. The rest are being dealt with over the phone.

What others have found

Heaney D and Gorman D (1996) Auditing out-of-hours primary medical care. *Health Bulletin.* **54:** 495–8.
Ten Midlothian practices in 1996 were visiting 63% of patients who made an out-of-hours request. Twenty-nine per cent of calls were dealt with by advice and 8% came to the surgery.

Salisbury C (1997) Observational study of a general practice out-of-hours cooperative: measures of activity. *BMJ.* **314:** 182–6.
Doctors from a London co-op in 1995 visited 32% of patients who telephoned the co-op. A commercial deputising service covering the same area visited 76% of patients and prescribed over a third more drugs than the co-op.

Jessopp L, Beck I, Hollins L *et al.* (1997) Changing the pattern out of hours: a survey of general practice cooperatives. *BMJ.* **314:** 199–200.
The median amongst the cooperatives surveyed was for 32% of phone calls to result in a home visit, 30% in attending a surgery and 38% in advice only.

Lattimer V, George S, Thompson F *et al.* (1998) Safety and effectiveness of nurse telephone consultations in out-of-hours primary care: randomised controlled trial. The South Wiltshire Out-of-Hours Project Group. *BMJ.* **317:** 1054–9.
Nurses managed 50% of calls without reference to a GP and reduced the need for both home visits and attendance at the primary care centre. There was no increase in the number of adverse events.

Salisbury C, Trivella M and Bruster S (2000) Demand for, and supply of, out-of-hours care from general practitioners in England and Scotland: observational study based on routinely collected data. *BMJ*. **320:** 618–21.

In 1997–98 in 20 English and Scottish co-ops the out-of-hours call rate (excluding bank holidays) was 159 per 1000 patients: 23.6% of calls resulted in a home visit, 29.8% in a centre consultation and 45.4% in telephone advice.

Hallam L and Cragg D (1994) Organisation of primary care services outside normal working hours. *BMJ*. **309:** 1593–4.

A survey of health authorities in 1993 found an average night visit rate of 35.7 per 1000 patients. In the main Northern cities it was higher at about 47 per 1000.

9 What is the link between consultation rates, deprivation levels and admission or referral to hospital?

What is the link between consultation rates, poverty and referrals to hospital? And do higher consultation rates in general practice lead to more or fewer hospital admissions or referrals? This chapter explores these questions using additional data from the Locality and Practice Information System (LAPIS) that has been run by Sheffield Health since 1994. LAPIS can be used to compare factors such as admission rates, referral rates, prescribing rates and deprivation levels across all Sheffield practices and the following clear conclusions can be drawn from this analysis:

- hospital admission rates and accident and emergency (A&E) attendance are higher in the more deprived parts of the city
- a practice with high admission rates will also tend to have high A&E admissions and, in a less clear-cut way, high referral rates.

It is also well documented that inner-city populations have more morbidity and social problems than those in the suburbs. Various large-scale studies based on the 1991/2 National Morbidity Survey of England and Wales have found a clear connection between the socio-economic status of individual patients and their consultation rate with a GP – poorer people tended to consult more often. We therefore expected GP activity rates to be part of an interconnecting web, influenced by deprivation and in turn influencing hospital attendance.

Bringing PDC data for 26 practices together with data from LAPIS for 1996 and 1997 sheds some further light on this complex interaction. A correlation analysis was undertaken using:

1   measures of GP activity, such as surgery consultations, daytime
    home visits, deputising service out-of-hours visits. (An initial
    analysis had indicated that nurse activity rates bore no relation-
    ship to anything.)
2   practice admission, referral and A&E attendance rates for
    Sheffield hospitals, plus practice prescribing levels and Town-
    send deprivation scores.

Practices with high GP consultation rates did show a weak
tendency to be in the more deprived parts of the city and to
have higher admission, referral and prescribing rates. However, the
relationships were mostly small enough ($r < 0.5$) that they could
have also been the result of chance variation. Further, the relationships could be attributed to a handful of practices who had high
levels of everything (GP contact, deputising service use, hospital
attendance and admission, deprivation and prescribing). Amongst
the other practices there was virtually no systematic pattern.

**The conclusion is that GP activity rates in Sheffield seem to be
only weakly related to measures of need or to activity in secondary
care.**

The lack of a major correlation between GP activity rates and the
LAPIS indicators is surprising. Other factors must be having a
greater effect. It was quite clear from the data, for instance, that
A&E attendance was affected by the proximity or otherwise of the
practice to the city's A&E department. Other factors may be
operating at an individual practice level. It may well be that the
type and quality of the service that a practice chooses to provide
has a crucial part to play in determining differences in activity rates
between practices. Such differences are not detectable simply by
looking at consultation rates.

GPs undoubtedly experience their surgeries as being driven by
demand. Precisely who comes through the door *is* principally
decided by the patients themselves. However it is likely that the
total amount of consultations is largely decided by the amount of
doctor time that the practice chooses to supply. A practice that is

accessible to patients in terms of opening hours and availability of appointments will have higher contact rates than a practice in the same area that has a more restricted access.

From the point of view of practices and PCG boards interested in what they could change, the following points emerge:

- differences in contact rates between practices are very hard to explain and almost certainly have more to do with history, personal styles and GP decisions about the quality of service to provide, than with demonstrable differences in demography or need
- whilst deprivation or morbidity may be an important governor of workload within some practices, at a PCG level it may well be hard to justify existing patterns of practice resource use (high *or* low) by reference to the demographic make-up of the practice populations.

This is frustrating since GPs and PCG boards will, understandably, seek some objective way of telling what the 'right' level of service to a particular population should be. In our view, a more profitable starting point than practice contact rates is measures of need that do not arise from within the practice. Examples might include:

- area (enumeration district preferably) based data about morbidity, mortality and, to an extent, deprivation. This could be for particular conditions such as coronary heart disease deaths and admissions
- countable populations that are known to have poor health or particular needs, e.g. drug users, the homeless and some ethnic minorities
- mismatches between known need and practice behaviour, e.g. small numbers of diabetics amongst practices with a high number of South Asians; low cardiology referrals in areas where coronary heart disease is rife.

Such an approach, however, requires sensitive and detailed data analysis. In urban areas patients can, and to some extent do, choose their GP on the basis of the type of service offered. For instance, two practices apparently drawing patients from the same disadvantaged population may have widely different numbers of ethnic minority patients, who may be disproportionately attracted to a GP of their own ethnicity. Or one practice may become known for taking on complex psychosocial problems whilst its neighbour explicitly adopts a narrower clinical definition of its role. Area-based data therefore needs to be interpreted in the light of local knowledge.

Further information

Further information can be found in our report:

- *The Missing Link?* December 1999.

Information about LAPIS can be obtained from Sheffield Health or from:

- Payne N, Jones G, Norris J *et al.* (1994) Profiling general practices. *British Journal of Healthcare Computing and Information Management.* **11**: 12–13.

Key points
- Aggregate GP contact rates in Sheffield seem to be only weakly related to measures of need or to activity in secondary care.
- Practice nurse contact rates bore no relation to measures of need or secondary care activity.
- The differences in GP contact rates between practices may be largely due to practice choices about the kind of service to provide.

What others have found

We know of no published study that has compared GP contact rates with referral and admission rates. However, there is a lot of evidence from elsewhere that social deprivation leads to higher contact rates with GPs for surgery consultations, daytime home visits and out-of-hours visits. It seems clear that *individual patients* are likely to consult more if they are poorer, unemployed, council tenants, from some ethnic minorities, etc. To some extent this translates through into *practices* working in more deprived areas having higher GP contact rates – but the relationship gets obscured by the differing approaches and styles of practices.

Carr-Hill R, Rice N and Roland M (1996) Socio-economic determinants of consultation in general practice based on the Fourth National Morbidity Survey of general practices. *BMJ.* **312:** 1008–13.
  The Fourth National Morbidity Survey showed that individual patients consult a GP more if they are unemployed, live in rented accommodation, live in an urban area (compared to rural area), are ethnically from the Indian sub-continent or live near the surgery.

Ben-Shlomo Y, White I and McKeigue P (1992) Prediction of general practice workload from census-based social deprivation scores. *Journal of Epidemiology and Community Health.* **46:** 532–6.
  The Third National Morbidity Survey showed that individual patients from lower socio-economic groups consulted GPs more than those in higher socio-economic groups.

Balarajan R, Yuen P and Machin D (1992) Deprivation and general practitioner workload. *BMJ.* **304:** 529–34.
  Data from the General Household Surveys for 1983–87 showed that GP consultation rates are higher in more deprived areas.

Balarajan R, Yuen P and Soni Raleigh V (1989) Ethnic differences in general practitioner consultations. *BMJ.* **299:** 958–60.
  General Household Survey data showed ethnic differences in GP consultation rates. People of Pakistani origin consulted more as did Indian and West Indian men.

Carlisle R and Johnstone S (1998) The relationship between census-derived socio-economic variables and general practice consultation rates in three town centre practices. *British Journal of General Practice.* **48**: 1675–8.
Patients living in the more deprived electoral wards had higher GP surgery consultation rates with these three Mansfield practices than those living in more affluent wards.

Aylin P, Majeed A and Cook D (1996) Home visiting by general practitioners in England and Wales. *BMJ.* **313**: 207–10.
The Fourth National Morbidity Survey showed that manual workers in social class V had nearly twice as many GP home visits as professionals in social class I – a much larger difference than in surgery consultations.

Carlisle R, Johnstone S and Pearson J (1993) Relation between night visit rates and deprivation measures in one general practice. *BMJ.* **306**: 1383–5.
The night visit rates of one large Mansfield practice were much higher from patients living in more socially deprived electoral wards than those living in more affluent parts of the town.

Carlisle R, Groom L, Avery A *et al.* (1998) Relation of out-of-hours activity by general practice and accident and emergency services with deprivation in Nottingham: longitudinal survey. *BMJ.* **316**: 520–3.
In six large Nottingham practices, both the out-of-hours contacts with the practice and with the hospital A&E department were significantly higher from patients living in more socially deprived electoral wards. General practice out-of-hours contacts and A&E rates were positively correlated (r = 0.5).

Majeed F, Cook DG, Hilton S *et al.* (1995) Annual night visiting rates in 129 general practices in one family health services authority: association with patient and general practice characteristics. *British Journal of General Practice.* **45**: 531–5.
Less than one-third of the inter-practice variation in night visiting rates in this London family health services authority (FHSA) could be explained by practice variations in age structure, chronic illness and social deprivation.

10 Is there a seasonal pattern to practice contact rates?

Every year there is media coverage of flu outbreaks and a winter surge in the demand for hospital beds. 'Common sense' would suggest that the demand to see GPs peaks in mid-winter, though the precise month might vary from year to year according to when the main flu outbreak struck. Does the data confirm this picture?

Figure 10.1 presents for an aggregate of 17 practices for three calendar years the monthly pattern of GP surgery consultations. Whilst there is some year to year variation, a certain broad pattern can be detected. August is a low consultation month whilst more generally the mid-summer to early autumn period has lower consultation rates than the winter, spring and early summer. However, the seasonal difference is far from dramatic, with rates in the highest month being only about 20% higher than the lowest month. Put another way, the month to month variation is no more than ±10%. That there is some tendency for higher rates in the winter can reasonably be attributed to colder weather generating more illness. There is, however, no sharp upsurge which could clearly be attributed to an influenza outbreak. The dip in August may be linked to patients' peak holiday time, though equally it may reflect that GPs are taking their holidays then and their surgeries are only partially being covered by locums.

Figure 10.2 presents comparable data for GP daytime home visits. GP home visit rates show a similar pattern to surgery consultations. August is just about the lowest month, with the peak occurring in December or January. Rates were generally lower in the summer and autumn compared to the winter and spring.

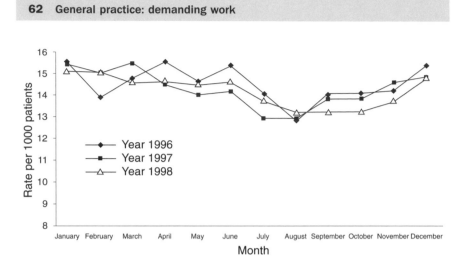

Figure 10.1:   GP in-surgery consultation rates per working day – 17 practices. The number of working days in each month in each calendar year was counted. Mondays to Fridays were counted as full days (except for bank holidays). Saturdays were counted as 0.1 of a day, based on the average number of consultations that took place during Saturday morning emergency surgeries.

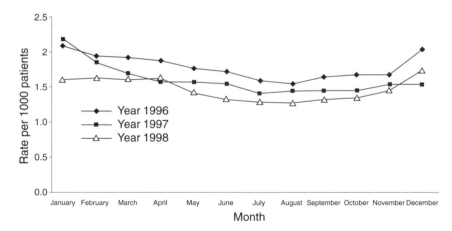

Figure 10.2:   GP daytime visit rates per working day – 17 practices. The same method was used as in Figure 10.1 for calculating the number of working days. The great majority of GP-undertaken daytime home visits will occur Monday to Friday, though some will occur at weekends.

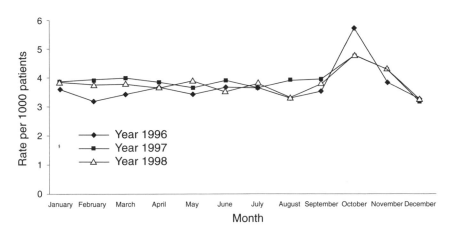

Figure 10.3: Practice nurse in-surgery consultation rates per working day – 17 practices.

However, the seasonal variation is greater, with rates varying ±20% from the average. The number of surgery consultations will be partly determined by the number of bookable appointments supplied. In comparison, the rate of home visiting is a purer measure of demand for a service.

Figure 10.3 presents the monthly consultation data for practice nurse surgery consultations. Here the seasonal pattern is very different. There is a clear peak in October, with some overspill into November. This will be due to the annual round of influenza vaccinations undertaken by practice nurses. Otherwise the monthly variation seems almost random. This is perhaps further evidence of consultation rates for practice nurses being governed by the supply of nurses and largely unrelated to patient demand.

Yet GPs and nurses *feel* that the workload in winter is harder. It *might* be the case that patients bring severer symptoms to the consultation in winter, though we have no data on that, and data presented in Chapter 12 shows that consultations are not any longer in the winter. The explanation may be a subjective one. Cold wet days, long hours of darkness and perhaps increased illness amongst health workers may leave them feeling that their work is harder.

Key points

- There is some tendency for GP contact rates to be higher in the winter and spring than in the summer and autumn. This is greater for home visits than for surgery consultations but is rather less than might have been expected.
- Practice nurse consultations show a clear peak in October due to the annual round of influenza vaccinations. Otherwise they show no seasonal pattern.

Making use of computer appointment data

Until this point our data analysis has been confined to aggregate contact rates. In Chapter 11 and many of the following chapters, we make use of comprehensive data on anonymised individual patients from the computer appointment systems and clinical systems of nine Sheffield practices.

The nine study practices were selected because they had the required computer software (either Meditel or Emis), including using a computer appointment system for all consultations.

From the computer appointment module, data was retrospectively extracted for every completed and uncompleted face-to-face consultation for any reason with either a doctor or practice nurse, occurring in the surgery premises during 1997 and 1998. This data included the date, who the consultation was with, and a patient number identifiable only within the practice. For one practice only, with about 7000 patients, comprehensive computer data was available on doctor visits during surgery opening hours only. The lack of data on home visits limits the relevance of this data in analysing the consultation patterns of the very elderly.

The consultation data was combined with information on patients from the practice clinical database. This was patient number, sex, age (in years), registration date, removal date (if left the practice), together with data on the presence of a clinical diagnosis, or the prescribing of particular medication during a time period, for a range of clinical conditions. No data that could identify any patient outside of the practice was collected. Temporary residents were excluded from the analysis. Miquest interrogation software was used to extract the data from the practices with Meditel. For the Emis practices it proved necessary to run a series of system-specific reports.

Data was collected for approximately 450 000 consultations and approximately 55 000 patients who were on the practices' list at some point during 1997 and 1998. Some analysis only took into account the patients who were on the list for the whole of the calendar year. The nine practices varied in size from 3600 to 7000 patients, and broadly reflected the range of Sheffield practices in terms of demographic structure and deprivation levels.

To test the validity of this data, the 1998 consultation history from the appointment module of 50 randomly selected patients in each practice was compared by practice staff with the best available alternative record. In some practices this was the Lloyd George continuation cards; in other 'paperless' practices this was the computer journal in the clinical database.

Neither record can be said to be the gold standard because continuation cards get separated from the main record, computer systems can be briefly shut down and clinicians sometimes fail to make an entry. However, 73% of records matched exactly, with a further 19% showing a discrepancy of only one consultation. Differences were distributed virtually evenly in both directions, so that in aggregate the appointment system recorded only 11 more consultations than the alternative record (1610 to 1599).

11 How long do patients have to wait to see a doctor?

Nothing perhaps irritates patients more than being told that there are no bookable appointments with a GP for several days. But how long do patients have to wait? And do they have to wait longer at certain times of the year?

Practices with computer appointment systems have a record of when each appointment was made and when it took place. The gap between the two is a measure of how long the patient waited for the appointment. However, the wait to see a GP is not simply analogous to a queue for a bus. Whilst many patients will want an appointment at the earliest opportunity, others will prefer to wait to see the GP of their choice who may only work part-time, be on holiday or be especially popular. Further, some appointments are initiated by the GP who, having seen a patient, asks them to make a further appointment for maybe one to four or even more weeks hence.

Figure 11.1 presents comprehensive data from the computer appointment system of seven Sheffield practices for all GP and practice nurse consultations in 1998. It shows what percentage of patients were seen on the same day, after one day through to 30 days:

- 35% of GP patients were seen on the same day as the appointment was requested, 65% were seen within three days of making the appointment and 85% within a week
- The figure also shows mini-peaks at seven, 14 and 28 days, reflecting patients coming back to see a GP 'in a fortnight'.

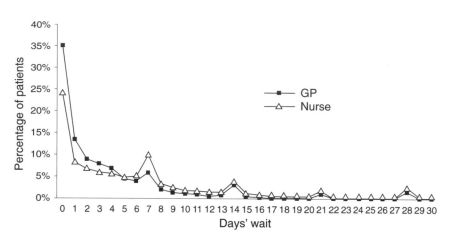

Figure 11.1: Days' wait for an appointment, 1998.

These peaks may underestimate the full amount of patients being recalled since a desire to see a GP 'in a week' may lead to a booking of an appointment for, say, six or eight days' time

• the percentages for 'seen within three days' and 'seen within one week' are similar to those recorded in the 1998 survey of NHS patients which was based on patient recall. However, in that survey only 13% of patients said they were seen the same day.

For practice nurses, the broad shape of the chart is similar to GPs but there are certain differences:

• fewer patient were seen on the same day – 25%
• fewer patients were seen within three days – 45%, and within a week – 70%
• relatively more patients were seen at seven, 14, 21 and 28-day intervals.

Practice nurses undertake more preventative work than GPs – screening, vaccinations, etc. – where they are inviting the patient to come in on a pre-set day. They also tend to work part-time and therefore to have clinics on certain days only, which may also be for particular conditions only. All this serves to explain both why patients wait longer to see them yet the 'wait to see a nurse' is rarely an issue.

A seasonal pattern?

If the demand for GPs was higher in winter this may lead to more GP consultations. However, if the supply of consultations is relatively fixed, an increase in demand could be expressed in the form of a hidden queue – that patients would have to wait longer to see the GP. Figure 11.2 explores this issue. It plots the average number of days' wait to see a GP for the seven practices in each month for both 1997 and 1998.

All appointments of 14 or more days' wait were excluded from this analysis on the assumption that the patient chose to wait that long rather than had to. A percentage of the appointments under 14 days' wait that were included in this analysis will similarly have been the result of patient choice. This analysis therefore tends to *overestimate* the wait to see a GP.

Figure 11.2 shows almost no seasonal pattern to the average number of days' wait. The sole exception is the drop in both years in December. Possibly this represents a slackening of demand over the holiday period, or perhaps it is a reflection that during the holiday period practices often resort to drop-in surgeries rather than offering pre-booked appointments.

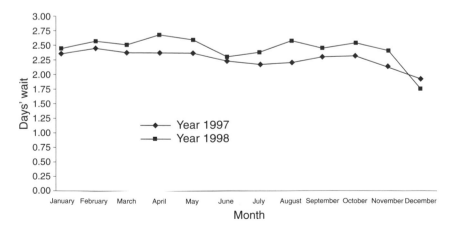

Figure 11.2: Average days' wait to see a GP.

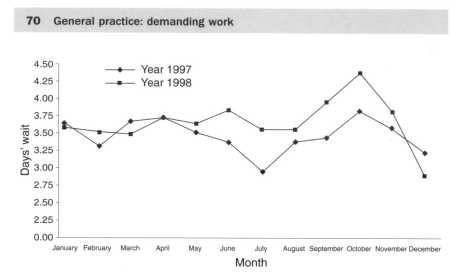

Figure 11.3: Average days' wait to see a practice nurse.

Figure 11.3 presents comparable data for practice nurses. This indicates a peak wait in October, which is probably due to nurses sending out lots of advance invites for influenza vaccinations. Otherwise there is little consistent pattern except for an equivalent drop to GPs in December.

Waiting times to see the doctor

Computer appointment systems record the time a patient arrives at the surgery, the time their appointment was due, the time the consultation began and the time it ended. Standard reports within some appointment systems can produce a record of waiting times. Table 11.1 compares the average result from five practices with a Meditel clinical system and the Front Desk computer appointment system for October 1998 with the results from the national survey of NHS patients in October 1998 which was based on the patient's memory of their last GP appointment.

More Sheffield patients were seen early or on time. This might be because the five practices are well organised. It might also be because patients tend to arrive early (on average 8.6 minutes early

Table 11.1: Comparison of waiting times to see a GP in the surgery		
	Five Sheffield practices October 1998	National NHS Survey October 1998
Early or on time	23%	7%
Late: less than 5 minutes	12%	11%
5–14 minutes	29%	42%
15–29 minutes	24%	25%
30–44 minutes	8%	8%
45 minutes +	4%	5%
Couldn't remember		2%

The Sheffield data is for all patients and had to be adjusted to match the time classification in the NHS survey. The national data is for adults only.

in the Sheffield data) and therefore tend to remember their wait from when they arrived rather than when their appointment was due.

Table 11.2 compares waiting times for GPs and practice nurses in the five Sheffield practices. For the nurses the month of September

Table 11.2: Comparison of waiting times to see a GP or practice nurse		
	GPs October 1998	Nurses September 1998
Early or on time	23%	27%
Late: 1–5 minutes	15%	16%
6–10 minutes	16%	16%
11–20 minutes	23%	22%
21–30 minutes	12%	9%
31–40 minutes	5%	4%
40 minutes +	6%	6%

Timings used are from the Front Desk computer appointment system.

is used because October would be atypical due to the influenza vaccination programme. There is a close fit between the two.

Further information

Further information can be found in our reports:

- *When can I see a doctor?* February 1997.
- *When is your next appointment? An exploration of general practice appointment systems,* September 1996.

Key points

- Thirty-five per cent of patients were seen by a GP on the same day as they made their appointment, 65% were seen within three days and 85% within a week.
- The equivalent figures for practice nurses were 25%, 45% and 70%.
- The wait to get an appointment with a GP or nurse showed little seasonal pattern.
- Thirty-five per cent of patients started their GP consultation within five minutes of its scheduled time, 64% within 15 minutes and 88% within 30 minutes.

What others have found

Kendrick T and Kerry S (1999) How many surgery appointments should be offered to avoid undesirable numbers of 'extras'. *British Journal of General Practice.* **49:** 273–6.

Analysis of the number of available appointments at the start of each day, and the number of extras who had to be fitted in, can help develop a formula for predicting the required number of appointments a practice needs to offer.

Marshall E (1986) Waiting for the doctor. *BMJ*. **292**: 993–5.

Shows how computer modelling based on a practice's own data can reduce patient waiting times by giving a more realistic appointment time.

Heaney D, Howie J and Porter A (1991) Factors influencing waiting times and consultation times in general practice. *British Journal of General Practice*. **41**: 315–9.

Data from 85 Lothian GPs showed large variations in consultation length and the time patients wait for the GP. Suggests strategies for reducing waiting times, such as having a mid-surgery break/catch-up time and tailoring the appointment system to individual GPs' consultation style.

Box 11.1:   The perfect appointment system?

Sadly, the perfect appointment system does not exist. Human beings, patients and GPs alike, are idiosyncratic. What works well for one set of GPs in one place will go wrong with different GPs and patients. But we do think there are some lessons to be learnt from both hard fact and qualitative experience – so, some suggestions:

- Computerise your appointment system. The computer packages that fit with different GP clinical systems vary in quality, but almost all clinicians and receptionists who use them find them more efficient than a paper system. They also provide comprehensive, routine data on consultations which you, or people like us, can analyse to improve your service.

- Good receptionists and practice managers have a feel for when demand is getting too great and extra appointments are needed. But analysis of past data (paper or computer) on seasonal patterns, weekly patterns and individual GP patterns can enable you to better predict the demand. We do not think sophisticated mathematical models are required, but a little data analysis can bear fruit.

- It would be nice to have a computer that sounded an alarm in the practice manager's office when the number of available advance appointments fell below a certain level. The technology and software is not there yet, but a practice could have a policy of checking its appointment book/ screen once a day. If, for instance, the number of appointments available on the following three days fell below a pre-set minimum level, consideration could be given to running another surgery.

- GPs usually run late, particularly by the end of the surgery. Patients get frustrated and take it out on receptionists. One solution is to have a planned short mid-surgery break in appointments to provide catch-up time, a chance of a coffee and perhaps even ten minutes with the other partners to exchange news.

- Another solution is to slightly lengthen the planned appointment time without lengthening it so much that it becomes common for the GP to be sitting waiting for patients. Computer modelling can help to work this out precisely, but pen and paper applied to some accurate computer appointment data on waiting times will do the job almost as well.

- GP consultation styles seem to be a very personal matter and very hard to change. A partnership argument about one GP consulting for too long is likely to still be an argument five years later. Perhaps the solution is to have different appointment lengths but an agreement that each doctor sees the same number of patients. Perhaps the long consulter is actually attracting patients with complex psychosocial problems that the other GPs are happy to be missing out on.

- In the last 15 years, general practice has swung heavily away from drop-in sessions to pre-booked appointments. Clinicians prefer the ability to predict and structure their workload. Many patients prefer it too, but a significant minority do not. An element of drop-in provision may have its place.

- Whether they are called drop-ins, extras or emergency appointments, a good quality appointment system has to preserve some planned space for urgent appointments generated by acute illness. Mostly these can be offered as short, one-problem-only consultations. But the system must not be rigid – not all acute illness is minor.

- The deeper issues are whether acute minor illness should be the work of GPs or practice nurses, **and** whether GPs should follow the example of many of their European and US colleagues and undertake more consultations by telephone or e-mail.

- Practices in poorer areas need to offer more consultations. Other things being equal, poor people have more illness and consult more than wealthier people.

- Some argue that the demand is potentially inexhaustible. There is no evidence to prove, or disprove, that belief but we do think that over the medium term demand responds to supply. Increase or reduce the supply of appointments and the number of appointments will, to some degree, go up or down accordingly. How else can we explain the phenomenon of neighbouring practices with similar types of patient having very different consultation rates?

- In the end, the number of appointments a practice provides is a quality issue. Here we define quality as a practice's opening hours; how long it is prepared to see patients wait for an appointment; whether its style of medicine is narrowly focused on a bio-medical approach or embraces a broad psychosocial approach; and *also* the quality of working life that its clinicians and receptionists have a right to expect. In the long run, burnt-out GPs are no good to anybody.

12 How long are GP and practice nurse consultations?

The appropriate length of a GP consultation has been the subject of much debate. Many have argued that longer consultations are a mark of quality, but pressure of numbers creates a strong pull towards short consultations. The historical trend has probably been towards longer appointment slots.

Patients with pre-booked appointments to see GPs and practice nurses are booked in at regular intervals. For GP surgeries these tend to be either 5, 7.5 or 10-minute intervals, though occasionally patients get a double appointment. Special clinics may have a longer appointment time such as 15 minutes, as may appointments for GP registrars in training. Nurse appointments tend to be longer, often 10 or 15 minutes, or even 20 minutes for a cervical smear, though appointments, if issued, for an influenza vaccination may be very short.

How does the reality match with the plan? The previous chapter indicated how GPs are usually running behind schedule, suggesting that on average they take a little longer than planned. A GP workload survey by the General Medical Services Council in 1992/3 found an average consultation time of 8.4 minutes, though this increased to 8.7 minutes if clinic appointments were included.

Table 12.1 presents selected results from seven Sheffield practices who provided comprehensive data on consultation length from their computer appointment system for the whole of 1998.

- The average GP consultation length was 8.9 minutes, but perhaps the biggest surprise was the almost identical nurse

Table 12.1:   Average length of consultation, 1998

Patient group	Doctor consultation	Nurse consultation
All	8.9	9.0
Male	8.6	8.7
Female	9.1	9.1
0–4 year-olds	7.1	7.7
5–14 year-olds	6.9	9.0
Adult range (10-year bands)	8.1–9.7	8.1–9.4
Inter-practice range	6.8–10.8	7.1–11.5
Individual practitioner range	5.3–12.2	7.1–13.9
Monthly range	8.6–9.4	9.0–9.6 (Oct. 6.7)
Locum doctors	7.7	
Registrars	12.2	
Patients with:		
diabetes	10.2	11.4
hypertension	9.5	8.8
chronic heart disease	10.0	8.9
asthma	9.0	9.1

The accuracy of this data depends on clinicians being consistent about when they switch their computer screen from one patient to another. Results for individual clinicians for 1998 were in fact fairly consistent with their data for 1997, suggesting that the data may be reasonably valid.

consultation time of nine minutes. A more detailed analysis showed that nurses had more very short consultations (partly for influenza vaccinations) and more longer consultations.

- The greatest source of variation was at the individual practitioner level, with a range from the fastest to the slowest for both GPs and practice nurses of about seven minutes. The inter-practice range was four minutes for GPs and 4.5 minutes for practice nurses.
- By contrast, the variation according to the type of patient was small. Women consulted for about half a minute longer.
- Consultations by children with GPs were about two minutes

shorter (which may be partly due to consultations for vaccinations), otherwise there was no consistent age pattern.

- Patients with chronic illness tended to consult for the average length of time once age differences were allowed for, though patients with diabetes seeing practice nurses showed a small tendency to longer consultations.
- There was no seasonal pattern, with the sole exception of nurse consultations in October which lasted only 6.7 minutes on average. This was because of the high number of short consultations for influenza vaccinations.
- Locum doctors tended to consult for a shorter time than GPs at 7.7 minutes, whilst registrars in training consulted for longer at 12.2 minutes.

Table 12.2 compares the Sheffield data with the results from the 1998 national NHS survey of patients' own perceptions of how long their last GP consultation took. The consultations in the Sheffield practices tended to be a little longer.

Table 12.2: Length of GP consultations with adults, 18 or over		
	Seven Sheffield practices 1998	National NHS Survey 1998
Less than 5 minutes	23%	23%
5–10 minutes	42%	53%
10–19 minutes	31%	21%
20+ minutes	4%	2%
Couldn't remember		1%

Are GP and practice nurse consultations really of equal length?

More detailed analysis of the Sheffield computer data indicated that GP surgeries tended to be an almost continuous flow of patients, whilst nurses often had gaps between seeing patients. This may reflect a less pressured schedule for nurses, but it may also partly reflect different consultation styles and roles.

GPs face a demand-led service in which they have to respond to patient pressure and move rapidly on to the next patient. This pressure encourages them to make each consultation as self-contained as possible. Many GPs will do any necessary note entries or other paperwork whilst the patient is in the room. Some develop a consultation style where they perhaps finish with the patient after seven minutes and then spend two minutes more on the paperwork. In either case, the aim is to contain the consultation within the allotted time.

The workload of practice nurses is more likely to be practice-initiated and to have a longer appointment slot. The detailed evidence from the practices studied here is that nurses seem, on average, to spend the same face-to-face time with the patient as the GP. However, they then complete all the necessary administrative work in a few minutes after the patient has left. Their face-to-face consultation time is therefore no longer than GPs.

Nursing studies have frequently reported that patients regard nurses as better at listening to them than GPs. This may be because they have the time to give the patient their full attention during their face-to-face contact.

Nurses and GPs also do different kinds of work: GPs provide much more acute medical care whilst nurses are more involved in chronic disease management or health promotion. Whether GPs' work should take more or less time than that undertaken by nurses is an open question. It may, arguably, also be the case that GPs, as the employer, receive more administrative support from their staff than do practice nurses.

Key points

- The main variation in consultation length is between individual practitioners and practices.
- By contrast, the type of patient makes little difference.
- GPs and practice nurses have very similar computer-logged average consultation lengths, though nurses have more very short *and* more long consultations than GPs.
- This may, however, mask a different consultation style, with GPs undertaking relevant administrative tasks *during* consultations and nurses *between* consultations.

What others have found

Howie J, Porter A, Heaney D *et al.* (1991) Long to short consultation ratio: a proxy measure of quality of care for general practice. *British Journal of General Practice.* **41**: 48–54.

Amongst 85 Lothian region GPs, consultations of ten minutes or more dealt with more relevant psychosocial problems, more long-term health problems and carried out more health promotion. Patients reported greater satisfaction with long consultations.

Williams M and Neal R (1998) Time for a change? The process of lengthening booking intervals in general practice. *British Journal of General Practice.* **48**: 1783–6.

Reports on the evidence for longer appointments. Details the process, results and benefits of changing from 7.5 to 10-minute appointments in a Yorkshire market town practice.

Hull FM and Hull FS (1984) Time and the general practitioner: the patient's view. *Journal of the Royal College of General Practitioners.* **34**: 71–5.

Some evidence that patient satisfaction improves when consultations are longer than 7.5 minutes.

Evaluation of nurse practitioner pilot projects, NHS Executive South Thames, Summary Report, November 1994.

Reports that patient satisfaction levels with GP consultations were high, but with nurse practitioners were higher still. Particular emphasis was given by patients to nurses' listening and empathising skills.

Doctors' and nurses' special issue. *BMJ (2000).* **320:** 1038–53.

Three randomised control trials of GP and nurse practitioner consultations all found longer consultation times for the nurses – between two and five minutes longer.

13 Who are GPs and practice nurses seeing?

In Appendix 1 we present charts from the 1991/2 National Morbidity Survey which show patient consultation rates by age and sex. Our analysis of detailed computer appointment data for nine Sheffield practices produced rates that were higher (particularly for practice nurses) but whose aggregate age–sex pattern of consultations was broadly similar. Such consultation rate charts based on age bands show the propensity of *individual* patients of different ages and gender to consult. Such rates do not take into account that the older age bands have fewer patients in them. The figures that follow take the perspective of the GP or practice nurse in terms of the number of consultations generated by patients of different gender and age groups. They are based on 1998 data, but an analysis for 1997 produced almost identical results.

Figure 13.1 presents the percentage of consultations with a GP by five-year age bands and by gender:

- amongst adults there were more consultations for women (60.8%) than men. This was particularly the case for younger women
- for both sexes, numbers of consultations in-surgery were lowest in older children/teenagers and the very elderly (though many of the latter will be seen at home by GPs)
- the highest number of consultations were with young women (but not young men). This will include consultations for contraception and maternity care
- the workload generated by men was spread fairly evenly across the age range.

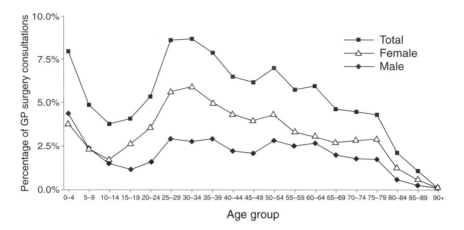

Figure 13.1: Percentage of GP surgery consultations by age group and gender, 1998.

Figure 13.2 presents the percentage of consultations with a practice nurse by five-year age bands and by gender:

- once again, amongst adults there were more consultations for women (63.5%) than men. This was particularly the case for younger women
- for both sexes, numbers of consultations in-surgery were lowest

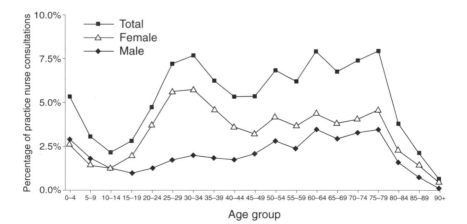

Figure 13.2: Percentage of practice nurse consultations by age group and gender, 1998.

in older children/teenagers and the very elderly (though some of the latter will be seen at home by some practice nurses)

- the highest number of consultations were with young women (but not young men). This will presumably be due to consultations for contraception, as well as cervical smears and other forms of well-woman consultation which also apply to middle-aged women
- numbers of consultations were relatively high for women and men in the 50–79 age range. This is presumably due to the nurses' role in chronic disease management and elderly assessments
- *individual patients* in the 50–79 age range consulted a nurse more often than younger adults, but the larger number of younger adults in the population means that nurses had nearly as many consultations with them as with the elderly.

Figure 13.3 compares the two patterns of GP and practice nurse surgery consultations. The pattern is similar, but with nurses seeing relatively more elderly people and GPs relatively more children and younger adults.

All nine practices had a broadly similar pattern of GP consultations by age and gender. What differences there were could partly

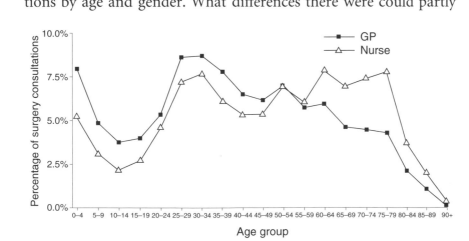

Figure 13.3: Percentage of surgery consultations by age group, 1998.

be explained by differences in the age–sex structure of their patient list. Who is seen by GPs is largely decided by the patients themselves, and it seems that aggregate patient behaviour is fairly similar from one practice to another.

For practice nurse consultations, however, there were some very large inter-practice variations. On average, females under 40 made up 39% of practice nurse surgery consultations, but this ranged from as low as 23% to as high as 57%. This is a reflection of practice nurses having very different roles. In one practice the supply of practice nurse appointments may be heavily geared towards contraceptive advice and well-woman clinics, in another they may be focused on chronic disease management amongst older people.

Figure 13.4 presents data for GP daytime home visits for the one practice that recorded such data on its computer appointment system. It shows that:

- over three-quarters (77.5%) of home visits were to women
- over two-thirds (68.2%) were to patients over 75
- 8% of visits were to women in the 25–39 age range, which presumably were related to maternity care

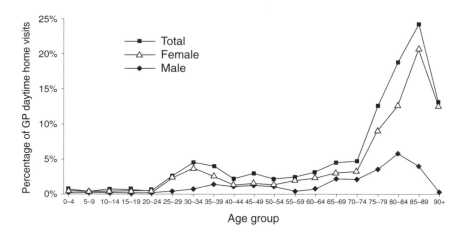

Figure 13.4:   Percentage of GP daytime home visits by age group and gender, 1998, one practice.

- whilst individual elderly men were less likely to be visited than women, the comparatively low number of visits to very elderly men is because men die at a younger age than women, so there are many fewer very elderly men.

We do not have such extensive data on the age–sex pattern of out-of-hours visits. However, a two-week survey of home visits in eight Sheffield practices in 1996 found a relatively even spread of visits across the age range, with a peak amongst children under five.

During surgery hours the demand for home visits will come from people who are unable to get to the surgery, and this will principally be elderly people whose illness will come on top of any pre-existing lack of mobility. Prior to the introduction of night surgeries at primary care centres, out-of-hours patients of all ages were in the same situation of not being able to attend for an urgent surgery consultation.

Key points

- Women consult GPs and practice nurses much more than men. This is particularly true amongst young women.
- A higher percentage of practice nurses' surgery consultations are with the elderly whilst GPs see relatively more younger people.
- There is much more inter-practice variation in practice nurse workload than there is for GPs.
- GP daytime home visiting is overwhelmingly to the over-75s, and particularly to elderly women.
- Out-of-hours visiting is more evenly spread across the population, with evidence for a peak in young children.
- Teenage boys and young men are a particularly difficult group to reach and special strategies may need to be adopted to provide effective care to high-risk subgroups. We have heard of one practice that has started running health promotion sessions in local pubs!

Comment: nursing homes

The rapid growth in nursing and residential home provision in the last ten years has given rise to a lot of concern amongst GPs that they are having to make many more visits to patients in these homes than they would to patients of a similar age living at home. It is not something that we have collected data on, but in the 'What others have found' section below we present the results of others' work.

What others have found

Jeffreys L, Clark A and Koperski M (1995) Practice nurses' workload and consultation patterns. *British Journal of General Practice.* **45:** 415–18.

Sixty-one per cent of practice nurse surgery consultations were by women in two inner-city practices. Peak demand was amongst women aged 25–34.

Aylin P, Majeed FA and Cook D (1996) Home visiting by general practitioners in England and Wales. *BMJ.* **313:** 207–10.

The Fourth National Morbidity Survey showed that GP home visiting was overwhelmingly to the over-75s. Visit rates varied from 103 per 1000 for people aged 16–24 through to 3009 per 1000 for those aged 85 and over.

Majeed F, Cook DG, Hilton S *et al.* (1995) Annual night visiting rates in 129 general practices in one family health services authority: association with patient and general practice characteristics. *British Journal of General Practice.* **45:** 531–5.

The percentage of the practice population aged under 15 was the most significant variable in explaining the variation in practice night visiting rates in one London FHSA.

Salisbury C, Trivella M and Bruster S (2000) Demand for, and supply of, out-of-hours care from general practitioners in England and Scotland: observational study based on routinely collected data. *BMJ.* **320:** 618–21.

In 1997/8 in 20 English and Scottish co-ops, the out-of-hours call rate was four times higher amongst children under five than for adults.

Carlisle R (1999) Do nursing home residents use high levels of general practice services? *British Journal of General Practice.* **49:** 645–6.
In one Mansfield practice, patients in nursing homes had nearly twice the number of GP contacts as patients over 74 living at home. Patients in residential homes were about halfway between the two. Ninety-nine per cent of contacts with nursing home patients were home visits compared to 48% for those at home.

Pell J and Williams S (1999) Do nursing home residents make greater demands on GPs? A prospective comparative study. *British Journal of General Practice.* **49:** 527–30.
The residents of eight Glasgow nursing homes had over twice as many GP contacts as elderly people living at home, though their consultations tended to be a little shorter.

McNiece R and Majeed A (1999) Socio-economic differences in general practice consultation rates in patients aged 65 and over: prospective cohort study. *BMJ.* **319:** 26–8.
The Fourth National Morbidity Survey showed that for people aged 65 and over, living in communal establishments or (to a lesser degree) living alone led to higher general practice contact rates and a greater demand for home visits than amongst those living at home with others.

Groom L, Avery A, Boot D *et al.* (2000) The impact of nursing home patients on general practitioners' workload. *British Journal of General Practice.* **50:** 473–6.
In nine Nottinghamshire practices, patients in nursing homes were compared with patients over 65 living in the community. The former had about three times more daytime home visits, out-of-hours visits and telephone calls than those in the community. The patients living at home visited the surgery far more often but overall the nursing home patients' GP contact rate was about 50% higher.

14 Defaulters in general practice: who are they and what can be done about them?

In general practice, as in the rest of the NHS, the attitude to patients who default on their appointment (Did Not Attends or DNAs) without giving prior notice is simple – defaulting is a bad thing and should be eliminated as far as possible. But is this best done by changing patient behaviour by education or punishment, or does it require changes in the appointment system? What does the evidence tell us?

We explored the aggregate pattern of default in nine Sheffield general practices, taking computer appointment data on 14 500 defaults in 1997. Six practices had the equivalent data for 1996 and three for 1995.

Table 14.1 presents the percentage of consultations in 1997 that ended in a default for various subgroups within the population. The 1996 data produced very similar results. The results for doctor consultations are in line with other studies in Britain and the USA.

- 68% of defaults occurred with a doctor, but the average default rate was higher with practice nurses (9.8% compared to 5.7%)
- for doctors, the default rate was highest among young adults, particularly 20–24 year-olds. For nurses, there were high default rates across the 0–34 age range
- 60.7% of all defaults were by women, but once the higher consultation rate of women was taken into account there was little gender difference in default rates
- GP default rates varied greatly between practices, and even more so for practice nurses. Default rates were clearly higher in the practices working in more deprived areas

Table 14.1:   Default rates, 1997

Subgroup	GP appointments	Practice nurse appointments
All patients	5.7	9.8
Practice range	3.0–13.0	1.6–19.2
Male	5.9	9.5
Female	5.5	9.9
0–4	3.9	14.1
5–14	5.0	16.6
15–24	11.5	16.7
25–34	8.8	13.9
35–44	6.2	10.1
45–54	4.4	8.2
55–64	2.7	5.4
65–74	2.2	4.2
75–84	2.8	5.7
85+	4.6	7.4
Same-day appointments	1.7	1.8
Next-day appointments	5.9	8.8
One-week appointments	8.6	12.6

- default rates showed little variation by day of the week or by time of the year
- default rates for same-day appointments were less than 2%. For next-day appointments they were 5.9% for GPs and 8.8% for practice nurses. There was a tendency for default rates to gradually increase the further in advance that the appointment had been made.

Figure 14.1 displays the age–sex default rates for GP appointments.

Frequent defaulters

Each year about 17% of patients defaulted on at least one appointment, but most of these defaulters (two-thirds) defaulted

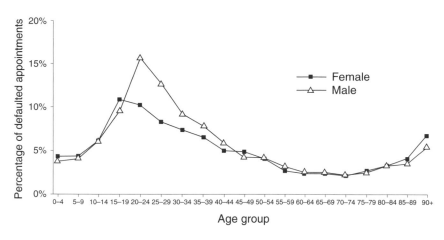

Figure 14.1:   GP in-surgery DNA rates, 1997.

once only. Seventy-five per cent of the once-only defaulters who remained on the practice list during the *following* year did not default again in that year. Thus most people who default only do it once and tend not to repeat the pattern.

A core of patients frequently defaulted: 1.2% defaulted more than three times per year, 0.35% more than five times per year. In both years these very frequent (more than five) defaulters were more likely to be women than men (60:40), with almost two-thirds aged 20–34. Of the 116 very frequent defaulters in 1996 who remained on the practice list throughout 1997, only 29 (25%) were very frequent defaulters in 1997. Patients who defaulted frequently also attended frequently: 60% of very frequent defaulters successfully attended ten or more appointments that year, and 90% were seen five or more times. Thus persistent defaulters are also persistent attenders, and only a quarter of frequent defaulters continued the behaviour in the subsequent year.

What can be done about defaults?

Many practices are concerned about their default rates and have tried reducing them using methods such as:

1 giving appointment cards to patients as reminders
2 signs in the waiting room outlining the problem and asking patients to turn up or ring to cancel
3 letters to frequent defaulters or a straight talking to by the GP.

Some have even suggested sanctions such as removal from the list or fining – though we do not advocate this.

Such approaches are based on changing patient behaviour and may have their place. If they work in your practice, or on some patients, that is fine. However, we know of no published study that has tested the effectiveness of such approaches in British general practice. Anecdotal evidence suggests mixed results, and that these methods are more likely to work in practices where the default rate is already comparatively low. Whilst our study cannot be definitive, it raises questions about the likely effectiveness of such approaches.

Most people defaulted once and did not repeat. Perhaps patients hear the educational messages from the practice. Alternatively, for most patients defaulting may be an exceptional occurrence which they are unlikely to repeat. They genuinely forgot, or they were unavoidably delayed.

A sizeable minority of defaults were caused by a small number of patients who both defaulted and attended frequently. Most ceased to be frequent defaulters the following year. It seems reasonable to assume that many were experiencing a life crisis of some form, or living a chaotic phase of their lives (they were mostly young people). They will have more pressing problems to deal with than their tendency to default. Focusing on the clinical management of the underlying problems is likely to be more effective in reducing the number of defaults of such patients than the use of administrative procedures to try and change their behaviour.

There may also be other approaches from the commercial sector which practices can adopt.

Some commercial organisations positively welcome defaulters since they give the opportunity to sell the same ticket twice. General practice lacks this financial incentive but practices with a default 'problem' might benefit from analysing their pattern of defaults to identify stable patterns, which they could then allow for by some selective overbooking of appointments.

For some people the problem of defaulters is simple: they waste GPs' time and cost the NHS money. In hospital out-patient clinics this may well be the case, but in general practice it is different. Generally speaking, GPs do not sit around waiting for patients to turn up – rather patients sit around waiting for GPs to catch up (as Chapter 11 demonstrated). For a harassed GP, a defaulted appointment can be a welcome breathing space. And the cost to the NHS of paying the GP or nurse will be the same, regardless of the default.

The people who really lose out from defaulted appointments are:

1   the patient who could have been seen that day but who was delayed because the appointment was blocked by the defaulter
2   in some cases the defaulter themselves – because they really needed to be seen.

If practices really want to avoid 'wasted' appointment slots then some limited and careful overbooking could be the answer. If, however, practices want to do their best to ensure that the defaulter actually turns up then a focus solely on the failings of the patient may not be sufficient.

Default rates are generally higher for nurse appointments. This is because rather more nurse than GP appointments are initiated by the practice – invitations for screening, health promotion, disease management, etc. The practice judges that this is for the patient's benefit but the patient clearly is not convinced. The practice may (or may not) be right but the patient has to be persuaded, or the appointment has to be better suited to their needs. Perhaps the invitation has to be done in a different way, the clinic run at a different time of day or the health check done opportunistically at a patient-initiated consultation. Equally, if patients are more likely to default on GP recall appointments, or on appointments made well in advance, this might indicate the need for changes in the way appointments are made. We are not advocating any particular technique, but rather a shift of focus from blaming the patient to redesigning the system.

Private enterprise aims to create a match between what customers want and what it is offering. It seeks to both change the customer by advertising methods and respond to customer preference. The phrase 'the customer is always right' is most definitely not a moral judgement but a pragmatic recognition of the best way to run a successful business in the long term.

Key points

- About 6% of GP and 10% of practice nurse appointments ended in a default.
- Default rates were found to be highest amongst young adults and, at a practice level, to be closely linked to deprivation.
- About two-thirds of those who defaulted only did it once during the year.
- A small core of patients defaulted very frequently, but only a quarter of these repeated their behaviour in the following year.
- The discussion suggests that strategies based on educating or punishing defaulters in order to change their behaviour may be of limited effectiveness.

Further information

Further information can be found in our report:

- *Did Not Attends: who are they and what can we do about them?* January 1999.

- Waller J and Hodgkin P (2000) Defaulters in general practice: who are they and what can be done about them? *Family Practice.* **17**: 252–3.

What others have found

Bickler CB (1985) Defaulted appointments in general practice. *Journal of the Royal College of General Practice.* **35**: 19–22.
GP default rates in one large practice varied from 7.2% to 14.6% according to the GP, and reached 18% for recall appointments. The longer the delay in getting an appointment, the higher the default rate. Defaults were more common at the end of the week.

Cosgrove M (1990) Defaulters in general practice: reasons for default and patterns of attendance. *British Journal of General Practice.* **40**: 50–2.
Reviews US studies on who defaulters in primary care are. Analyses reasons for default in 40 patients in a Leeds practice, the principal reasons being too ill to attend, symptoms resolved and forgot the appointment time.

15 Frequent attenders: who are they?

The average patient sees a GP or practice nurse in the surgery premises about four times a year. However, some patients consult much more frequently than this, up to an extreme of 77 consultations a year in this analysis. Who are these frequent attenders?

The results presented here are based on an analysis of comprehensive computer appointment data from nine Sheffield practices for 1998. An analysis for 1997 produced very similar results. A limitation of this analysis is that it takes no account of home visits since eight of the nine practices did not record home visits on computer. For most of the age range, home visits are such a tiny percentage of consultations as to be irrelevant, but for elderly patients this is not the case.

A pragmatic definition of frequent attenders was used: patients who were seen in surgery 20 or more times per annum by either a GP or practice nurse. These comprised **1.3% of the patients** of the nine practices studied, but they generated **8.3% of the consultations**. The inter-practice variation around the average was from 0.3% to 2.0%. There was also a major variation by age. Only 0.1% of children aged 5–14 were frequent attenders, whilst amongst adults aged 60–69 the rate was almost 2.5%. Lowering the frequent attendance threshold to 15 or more consultations showed that 3.6% of patients generated 17.6% of consultations. Frequent attenders are clearly few in number but contribute significantly to practice workload.

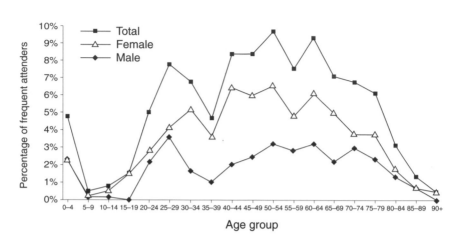

Figure 15.1: Percentage breakdown of patients attending surgery 20 or more times, 1998.

What age and sex are frequent attenders?

Figure 15.1 looks at the numbers of patients who consulted a doctor or practice nurse in-surgery 20 or more times during 1998. It presents this by five-year age bands as a percentage of the total number of frequent attenders (602). Frequent surgery attenders were principally middle-aged adults. They were also more likely to be women, by a ratio of about 2:1. This mirrors the well-documented tendency for women in the 15–70 age range to consult more than men. Data from the one practice that entered home visits on computer indicated that including home visits increased the number of elderly frequent consulters but had no effect in the rest of the age range.

Do frequent attenders have a lot of chronic illness?

One would expect frequent attenders to have more illness than patients who attend less. Figure 15.2 explores this issue. Data was

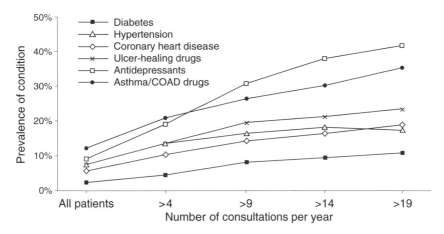

Figure 15.2: Prevalence of condition according to number of surgery consultations, 1998.

collected from the practices on the prevalence of a number of common long-term illnesses. These were diabetes, treated hypertension, coronary heart disease (CHD) and patients receiving ulcer-healing drugs, antidepressants and medication for asthma or chronic obstructive airways disease (COAD). (For more details of this study, *see* Chapter 17.)

The left-hand corner of Figure 15.2 shows the prevalence of each condition amongst the whole patient population. As the population base is narrowed to those patients with more than four, nine, 14 and 19 consultations, the prevalence of all the conditions progressively increases. Thus 9% of the population studied had received a script for an antidepressant during 1998, but amongst those patients who had attended more than 19 times the prevalence was 42%. Overall, patients who attended on more than 19 occasions were three to four times more likely to have a chronic condition than the average patient. This is clear evidence that many frequent attenders have some long-term illness.

However, this should be tempered by the fact that 22% of patients with more than 19 attendances had none of the above conditions. It is also worth noting the high prevalence of patients on antidepressants amongst frequent attenders. These facts fit with other research that suggests that frequent attendance often cannot be explained on grounds of morbidity alone and that frequent attenders are likely to have psychosocial problems.

Are frequent attenders the same people from year to year?

Data was available for all nine practices for 1997 and 1998, for six for 1996 and for two for 1995. It was therefore possible to track the attendance pattern of individuals from year to year via their internal practice number.

Of those patients with more than 19 attendances who remained at the practice during the following year, about one-third were frequent attenders in the subsequent year. This closely matches other research. The conclusion is that there is a hard core of people who go on attending frequently each year, but that these are less than half of all frequent attenders. The remainder may, in part, be people who are experiencing a life crisis of some form which within a year is resolved.

What can be done about frequent attendance?

Since frequent attenders generate such a high percentage of GP workload, it is important to ascertain whether this is time well spent. Where frequent attendance is based on chronic physical illness, the question can reasonably be asked whether these patients should be seeing a GP or a practice nurse.

For frequent attenders with mental illness or psychosomatic complaints, a number of studies suggest that these patients' symptoms do not require psychiatric intervention. However, treatment by a counsellor, or by a therapist and GP working together, may be more effective than repeated consultations with a GP. Various current studies are being undertaken nationally to explore this question.

Further information

Further information can be found in our report:

• *Frequent Attenders: who are they?* September 2000.

Key points

• 1.3% of patients generated 8.3% of all surgery consultations.
• Two-thirds of frequent attenders were women, and frequent surgery attenders tended to be middle-aged.
• Frequent attenders were much more likely to have a chronic physical illness than other patients, and 42% were taking antidepressants.
• About one-third of frequent attenders repeated their behaviour in the following year.

What others have found

Aylin P, Majeed FA and Cook D (1996) Home visiting by general practitioners in England and Wales. *BMJ.* **313**: 207–10.
    The Fourth National Morbidity Survey showed that 1.3% of patients had five or more visits per year from their GP, and 0.3% had ten or more. This constituted 39% and 17% respectively of all home visits.

Gill D, Dawes M, Sharpe M *et al.* (1998) GP frequent consulters: their prevalence, natural history and contribution to rising workload. *British Journal of General Practice.* **48**: 1856–7.
    Two-thirds of frequent consulters in an Oxford practice were female. Only one-third of frequent consulters repeated their behaviour in

the following year. However, over a five-year follow-up, 75% of frequent consulters repeated their behaviour in at least one other year.

Baez M, Aiarzaguena J, Grandes G *et al.* (1998) Understanding patient-initiated frequent attendance in primary care: a case-control study. *British Journal of General Practice.* **48**: 1824–7.
Older patients in nine Spanish general practices were more likely to be frequent attenders. Sixty-one per cent of frequent attenders had a chronic physical illness, 51% had a mental disorder and 20% were exposed to high life stress. These three factors plus age explained 82% of frequent attendance.

Neal R, Heywood P, Morley S *et al.* (1998) Frequency of patients consulting in general practice and workload generated by frequent attenders: comparison between practices. *British Journal of General Practice.* **48**: 895–8.
Seventy-five per cent of frequent attenders were women, and older patients were over-represented in four Leeds practices: 1% of patients generated 6% of consultations, 3% generated 15% of consultations, 20% generated 55% of consultations and 50% generated 90% of consultations.

Heywood P, Blackie G, Cameron I *et al.* (1998) An assessment of the attributes of frequent attenders to general practice. *Family Practice.* **15**: 198–204.
In one large practice, 86% of very frequent attenders (15+ GP consults) were female and 94% had a chronic physical or mental health problem. Compared to controls they had five times the level of prescriptions and referrals.

Vedsted P and Olesen F (1999) Frequent attenders in out-of-hours general practice care: attendance prognosis. *Family Practice.* **16**: 283–8.
In Aarhus, Denmark in 1990, 10% of the most frequent users of the out-of-hours service made 42% of the contacts. One-third of frequent attenders repeated their behaviour the following year, and 7% repeated it in all the following four years.

Larivaara M, Vaisanen E and Wynne L (1996) Developing a family systems approach to rural healthcare: dealing with the 'heavy user' problem. *Families' Systems and Health.* **14**: 291–302.

Fifty-four per cent of heavy users of general practice in a rural Finnish community had psychosomatic symptoms or disorders compared to 24% with chronic physical disorders. However, few had psychiatric disorders or a history of psychiatric treatment. Proposes family-oriented treatment with collaboration between GPs and family therapists.

Dowrick C, Bellon A and Gomez M (2000) GP frequent attendance in Liverpool and Granada: the impact of depressive systems. *British Journal of General Practice.* **50**: 361–5.

Depressive symptoms were by far the major predictor of frequent attendance in two practices in England and Spain.

16 Do newly registered patients consult more frequently?

Practices where a high percentage of patients join and leave each year usually believe that this adds to their workload. Is this true?

Responding to the needs of new patients includes undertaking new patient checks, for which the practice receives an item-of-service payment (£7.80 in 1999). However, new patients may create extra work in other ways which do not lead to any additional financial reimbursement. If they have moved house they may not register with a GP until they have an urgent medical problem, and responding effectively to someone whose medical history and family background is unfamiliar may demand extra time.

A few practices will have a high turnover because of a large student population. They may therefore do many new patient checks, yet this will be compensated for by them having a young and healthy population. For other practices, high turnover may be due to serving unpopular council estates or having many refugees and asylum seekers, and for them the consequent extra workload could be quite demanding.

To explore this question we analysed data from the computer appointment systems of nine Sheffield practices with a combined list size of about 50 000 patients, looking at the in-surgery consultation record of every patient who joined the list in 1997.

Method

Turnover was defined here as the number of patients joining the list during a calendar year divided by the average list size of the practice. Seven of the practices had 'average' for Sheffield turnover rates for new patients in the 6.5–9.5% range. Two had high rates of about 15%. One of these served an unpopular council estate and the other a more affluent area with many young people in their twenties. None had very low rates.

Nearly 5000 patients joined the list of these nine practices during 1997 and Figure 16.1 shows the age range as percentages of the total. Ten per cent of new patients were newborn babies. These clearly present a very different kind of workload to other types of new patient and they were excluded from this analysis. The highest percentages of new patients were amongst young adults and children aged one to four. This represents young people leaving home and young families moving to a new house.

For all new patients, the number of in-surgery consultations (with either a doctor or a practice nurse) was counted for both their first three months with the practice and for the subsequent three months. New patients who left the list during that time were not counted in the analysis. The three-monthly consultation rates for new patients were then compared with the average three-monthly consultation rate of pre-existing patients (those who were on the list on January 1st 1997 and remained so for the whole year).

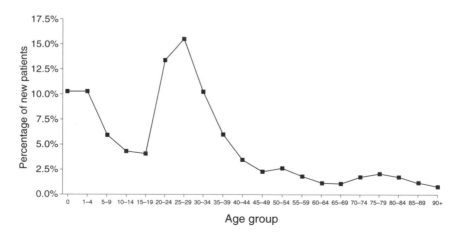

Figure 16.1: New patients by age group as a percentage of all new patients, 1997.

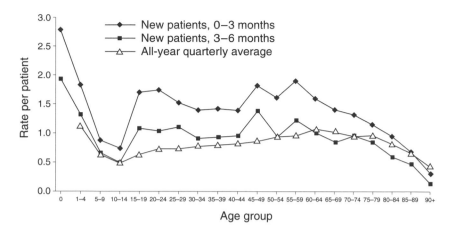

Figure 16.2:   GP in-surgery quarterly consultation rates, 1997.

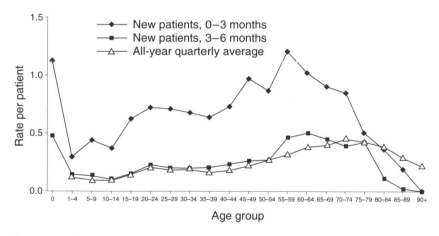

Figure 16.3:   Practice nurse in-surgery quarterly consultation rates, 1997.

Figures 16.2 and 16.3 present the results plotted by five-year age groups. Babies under one year were treated separately from those aged one to four years because all babies under one are 'new' patients and so there is no pre-existing group to draw comparisons with. Babies were therefore excluded from the analysis that follows.

Results

- Figure 16.2 shows that for almost the entire age range, new patients in their first three months on the list consulted a doctor more frequently than the quarterly average for pre-existing patients of the same age. On average they had an **extra 0.6 consultations**.
- The exception was in the over-75s where there was no evidence of extra consultations. However, in the very elderly many consultations take place in the patient's home and this data was not available from the computer appointment system.
- During their second three-month period on the list, the consultation rate had fallen across the entire age range and was now close to the average consultation rate of pre-existing patients at only **0.16 consultations extra**.
- Figure 16.3 shows the equivalent rates for in-surgery consultations with practice nurses. Once again, new patients in their first three months consulted markedly more than pre-existing patients, except among the over-75s. This amounted to an **extra 0.4 consultations**.
- During their second three-month period on the list, the consultation rate for new patients had fallen across the entire age range to become little different from the pre-existing patient average.

Combining doctor and nurse consultations produces a figure of **1.16 extra surgery consultations for each new patient**.

To understand practically what these figures mean, compare three practices each with a list of 5000:

Practice A has a low turnover of 3% (i.e. 150 new patients per year).
Practice B has a relatively average turnover of 8% (i.e. 400 new patients per year).
Practice C has a high turnover of 13% (i.e. 650 new patients per year).
* All excluding newborn babies.

This study predicts that Practice B would have 304 extra doctor consultations and 160 extra nurse consultations during the year. Put another way, this amounts to just under two extra consultations in-surgery each weekday. This amounts to about 2% of an average practice's consultation workload. This figure is not trivial, but neither can it be said to constitute a major governor of practice workload.

Comparing practices A and C, the latter would have 380 more doctor consultations and 200 more nurse consultations per year than the former. This amounts to a 2.2% higher doctor consultation rate and a 4.3% higher nurse consultation rate than practice A.

More detailed analysis showed that of all the consultations by new patients in their first three months, 21% of nurse consultations and 12% of doctor consultations occurred on the day of registration. Thereafter the weekly consultation rate slowly declined from a week one peak until it stabilised from about week 19 onwards. This initial peak could be due to two factors:

- new patients registering because they have an immediate problem which needs sorting out
- practices asking patients to have a 'new patient check' at the time of registration.

How many of the extra new patient consultations were generated by the reimbursable new patient checks was outside the scope of this analysis. Clearly, not all new patients have such checks, but data was not available on whether the percentage is, say, 50% or 75% (which would mean an extra 0.5 or 0.75 consultations per patient per year). In the absence of such data it seems reasonable to surmise that virtually all the extra nurse consultations were due to new patient checks but these were only a part of the extra doctor consultations.

Further information

Further information can be found in our report:

- *New Patients: does a high turnover create extra work?* September 1999.

Key points

- On average, new patients had 0.76 extra GP consultations and 0.4 extra practice nurse consultations compared to pre-existing patients, and these occurred during their first four months on the practice list.
- For a practice with an average patient turnover, the extra consultations generated by new patients amount to about 2% of its consultation workload.

---

17 What is the effect of long-term illness on consultation rates?

To state the obvious, people visit their GP because they are ill. We would therefore naturally expect people with long-term illnesses such as diabetes, coronary heart disease or asthma to visit their GP more often than somebody who does not have the condition. But by how much more? And is their condition being managed by doctors or nurses?

The 1991/2 National Morbidity Survey contains such information, but it tends to be buried in detailed tables. It is also now nearly 10 years old and a lot has changed in the way chronic illnesses such as diabetes and asthma are treated in general practice, particularly the role of practice nurses. Whilst some 'paperless' practices now directly enter the reason for every consultation into their computer database, this is still a small minority and extracting the data for analysis is generally far from easy.

We wanted to develop a method of measuring the workload associated with different chronic illnesses, for both GPs and practice nurses, that could be based on routinely collected data but did not rely on practices being committed data recorders. In doing so we made use of nine practices' complete appointment data for 1997 and 1998, combined with information from the clinical database on various long-term illnesses. The practices had either Meditel or EMIS systems. The findings are based on an analysis of about 450 000 consultations.

Box 17.1: Statistician's health warning

We've tried to present some relatively complex ideas, assumptions and methods in a fairly simple way. If you still find there is more statistics than you are comfortable with, you can always jump to the key points at the end. Those who want more detail and statistical robustness will need to get a copy of our full report on this work – *Looking After Long-term Illness: implications for practice consultation rates*, October 1999.

Clinical conditions

The conditions chosen for study were commonly occurring long-term illnesses that were expected to generate significant numbers of consultations, and which it was felt could be identified on an average practice's computer record by clinical coding and/or drug regime.

The precise definition used for each condition is specified in Table 17.1. The definitions are entirely pragmatic, being based on evidence of a diagnosis and/or prescribing.

Definitions wholly or partly based on drug regime used the presence of *one* prescription during the year as an indicator. This is comparable with other research. A *two or more* prescription definition might have been preferable but in practices using the EMIS computer system this data could not be obtained. Using only one prescription per year increased the prevalence of people selected as having the condition by about 30% and probably picked up people with a milder version of the condition, as well as some who may not have had it at all. Analysis of those people selected using a two-script definition showed that their consultation rates were a little higher than those selected using a one-script definition. This means that the consultation rates

Table 17.1: Definitions of clinical conditions studied

Condition	Definition
Diabetes	A diagnosis of diabetes mellitus in the computer record.
Hypertension	A diagnosis of hypertension in the computer record *and* with a prescription for any of the following drugs during that year: thiazide or loop diuretics, beta-blockers, ACE inhibitors or calcium-antagonists.
Coronary heart disease	A diagnosis of CHD in the computer record *or* with a prescription for a nitrate during that year.
Taking medication for peptic ulcers	A prescription on computer for a drug in *British National Formulary (BNF)* category 1.3 – ulcer-healing drugs – during that year.
Taking medication for depression	A prescription on computer for a drug in *BNF* category 4.3 – antidepressant drugs – during that year.
Taking medication for psychosis*	Aged under 60 and with a prescription on computer for a drug in *BNF* category 4.2 – drugs used for psychoses and related disorders – during that year.
Taking medication for asthma	Aged under 40 years and with a prescription on computer for any of the following drugs during that year: beta$_2$ adrenoceptor stimulants, inhaled corticosteroids or asthma prophylactics.
Taking medication for chronic obstructive airways disease	Aged 40 years or over and with a prescription on computer for any of the following drugs during that year: beta$_2$ adrenoceptor stimulants, other bronchodilators, inhaled corticosteroids or asthma prophylactics.

* Only people under 60 were included in this definition because in the elderly some of these drugs can be used to treat dementia and confused states.

presented in this study for people with long-term illness are likely to err on the side of being too low.

In all conditions the pattern of prevalence by age and sex conformed to both that found in the 1991/2 National Morbidity

Survey, and published data from the Department of Health's General Practice Research Database for 1994–1996. However, the scale of prevalence was consistently 50–100% higher than the NMS and 33–50% higher than the GPRD. Much of this difference will be due to the different definitions used. However, some may be real, perhaps due to urban Sheffield having more chronic illness than the national average, or to an increase in chronic illness since 1991. The study prevalence for diabetes, hypertension and coronary heart disease was similar to that found in the 1994 Health Survey for England.

Results

An initial analysis was undertaken to compare both the doctor and practice nurse in-surgery consultation rates of patients with a single condition to the much larger number of patients without the condition. Comparison was made by ten-year age bands.

Figures 17.1 and 17.2 present the results for all nine practices for patients with and without diabetes in 1998. The doctor consultation rate is significantly higher for those with diabetes except

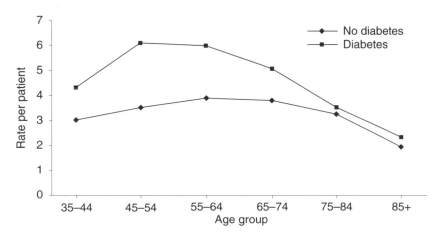

Figure 17.1:   GP in-surgery consultation rates, 1998 – diabetes.

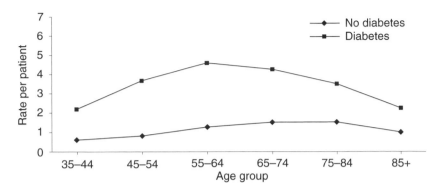

Figure 17.2:   Practice nurse in-surgery consultation rates, 1998 – diabetes.

amongst the very elderly. For practice nurses the difference is even greater.

Figure 17.3 presents the results for doctor consultations for patients taking antidepressants. Compared to diabetes the excess of consultations is much greater, though once again the gap narrows sharply amongst the elderly. The results for the one practice with home visit data showed a marked excess of doctor consultations (in surgery plus at home) across the entire age range, with no drop off in the very elderly. For practice nurses the

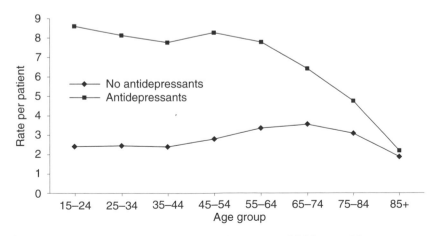

Figure 17.3:   GP in-surgery consultation rates, 1998 – antidepressants.

difference in consultation rates between the two groups was small, though still statistically significant in the under-65s.

The results for all the conditions studied for doctor consultations were a variation on this common theme of marked and statistically significant differences, though only hypertension and CHD were significant in the 85+ age range. For nurse consultations there were statistically significant differences in consultation rate for every condition except patients taking antipsychotic medication. However, the scale of difference varied greatly between conditions. An identical analysis for 1997 produced very similar results. The broad pattern of extra consultations with doctors and nurses for each clinical condition also held true at an individual practice level.

Tables 17.2 and 17.3 present the average consultation rates with doctors in-surgery by sex, condition and ten-year age bands for 1998. Also presented are the consultation rates for all patients and for patients who had none of the conditions studied.

The analysis presented so far shows how often people who have a particular long-term condition and are of a certain age and sex consulted on average. It also shows how often people of the same age and sex who do not have the condition consulted. It does not directly tell us *why* people consulted. Rather an inference is made that the *extra* consultations are wholly or partly to do with the person's chronic condition.

Are the extra consultations associated with long-term illness distributed evenly or unevenly by gender? For those people taking medication for asthma, COAD, ulcers or depression, the extra consultations were fairly evenly distributed between men and women. For diabetes, hypertension and CHD there were more extra consultations per person by men in a ratio of broadly 3:2. These patterns largely held for both doctor and nurse consultations, and for 1997 as well as 1998. For people taking antipsychotic medication, women had more extra consultations with doctors than men, also in a ratio of 3:2, but there was little difference in nurse consultations.

Table 17.2: Average doctor in-surgery consultation rates, 1998 (females)

Condition	Age 0–4	5–14	15–24	25–34	35–44	45–54	55–64	65–74	75–84	85+	All ages (average)
Diabetes	–	–	–	–	5.35	6.98	6.67	5.63	3.51	2.45	5.04
Hypertension	–	–	–	8.95	5.70	6.44	5.74	5.18	4.04	2.50	4.93
Coronary heart disease	–	–	–	–	–	8.59	7.68	5.86	4.21	2.50	5.28
Ulcer-healing drugs	–	–	7.86	7.38	7.66	8.26	7.56	6.58	4.93	2.34	6.52
Antidepressants	–	–	9.18	8.64	8.25	8.82	8.14	6.46	4.61	2.19	7.51
Antipsychotics	–	–	–	11.42	9.39	10.32	8.26	–	–	–	10.11
Asthma drugs	6.56	3.89	5.54	6.52	6.78	–	–	–	–	–	5.63
COAD drugs	–	–	–	–	7.52	7.75	7.15	6.37	4.83	2.08	6.43
No condition	3.50	1.89	2.99	3.21	2.74	2.90	2.74	2.47	1.92	1.21	2.71
All patients	3.89	2.26	3.67	4.15	3.89	4.41	4.54	4.26	3.27	1.89	3.75

Rates are not shown where there were less than 20 people in the age–sex band.

Table 17.3: Average doctor in-surgery consultation rates, 1998 (males)

Condition	Age 0–4	5–14	15–24	25–34	35–44	45–54	55–64	65–74	75–84	85+	All ages (average)
Diabetes	–	–	–	–	3.30	5.41	5.55	4.63	3.57	2.00	4.48
Hypertension	–	–	–	4.24	4.61	4.85	4.97	5.07	4.02	3.20	4.72
Coronary heart disease	–	–	–	–	4.90	5.85	5.59	5.10	4.12	2.76	4.93
Ulcer-healing drugs	–	–	5.46	5.27	5.58	5.62	5.83	5.75	4.87	2.73	5.46
Antidepressants	–	–	7.40	7.04	6.88	7.15	7.18	6.53	5.25	2.36	6.74
Antipsychotics	–	–	–	9.45	5.66	5.61	5.55	–	–	–	6.79
Asthma drugs	–	3.29	3.36	4.14	4.57	–	–	–	–	–	4.08
COAD drugs	–	–	–	–	4.76	5.44	5.98	5.73	4.65	2.96	5.35
No condition	3.63	1.62	1.42	1.40	1.41	1.66	2.06	1.89	2.11	1.94	1.69
All patients	4.19	1.97	1.77	1.95	2.14	2.65	3.44	3.52	3.42	2.28	2.52

Rates are not shown where there were less than 20 people in the age–sex band.

Co-morbidity

Many people with one major condition also have other major diseases. If such co-morbidity is common, the results presented above could be partially misleading. Given for instance that 30% of people with diabetes had hypertension and 28% had CHD, what is the independent effect of each condition on patient consultation rates? Table 17.4 shows the average doctor consultation rate for people with the condition (not allowing for age or sex) and then the average rate for those with two conditions. Co-morbidity is shown where more than 25% of people with the first condition also had the second.

In every case, those people with co-morbidity had a higher consultation rate than those with just one of the conditions. The combined consultation rates are less than would be obtained by simply adding together the extra consultations for each condition.

Table 17.4: Average doctor in-surgery consultation rates, 1998			
People with/taking	Consult. rate	Co-morbidity	Consult. rate
No condition	2.19		
All patients	3.15		
Diabetes	4.75		
		Diabetes + hypertension	5.26
Hypertension	4.85	Diabetes + CHD	5.62
		CHD + hypertension	5.55
Coronary heart disease	5.10		
		CHD + ulcer-healing drugs	6.55
Ulcer-healing drugs	6.04		
		Ulcer-healing drugs + antidepressants	8.28
Antidepressants	7.28		
		Antipsychotics + antidepressants	10.46
Antipsychotics (<60)	8.53		
Asthma drugs (<40)	4.77		
COAD drugs (40+)	6.00		

This is presumably because people with two problems may bring them both to the same consultation.

To further explore the effect of co-morbidity we used the statistical technique of multiple regression analysis. This provided a sophisticated mathematical way of measuring the effect on consultation rates of each condition, taking into account the effects of all the other conditions and differences in age and sex. For statistical reasons the analysis had to be done across the entire age range so the data on people under 60 taking anti-psychotics was excluded, whilst asthma in the under-40s and COAD in the over-40s were combined into one all-ages asthma/COAD variable.

The results for 1997 and 1998 are presented in Table 17.5. The 'regression coefficients' effectively represent the *extra* consultations per person per year attributed by the statistical model to the presence of the condition, having allowed for the effect of all the other variables.

Comparison of columns A and B of Table 17.5 shows that for diabetes, practice nurse consultations outnumbered GP consultations by nearly 4 to 1. By contrast, for all the other conditions

Table 17.5: Results of multiple regression analysis

| Condition | Regression coefficients | | | |
	(A) Doctor consultations 1998	(B) Practice nurse consultations 1998	(C) Doctor consultations 1997	(D) Practice nurse consultations 1997
Diabetes	0.62	0.92	2.32	2.16
Coronary heart disease	0.99	1.27	0.48	0.31
Hypertension	1.12	1.35	0.79	0.65
Ulcer-healing drugs	1.92	1.99	0.17	0.15
Asthma/COAD drugs	2.04	2.23	0.50	0.50
Antidepressants	3.60	4.14	0.18	0.26

the majority of extra consultations occurred with the doctor. For coronary heart disease for instance the extra doctor consultations were twice the number of practice nurse consultations, whilst for patients taking antidepressants the equivalent ratio was 20 to 1.

The rates for 1997 for both doctors and nurses are broadly similar to 1998, though the differences are enough to indicate that the figures on extra consultations presented here should be seen only as *rough estimates*.

Table 17.6 presents for 1998 the extra workload generated by the different conditions per 1000 patients on the practices' list, taking into account the actual prevalence of the condition on the list. It shows, for instance, that CHD generated comparatively few extra consultations per 1000 patients (56 for doctors, 27 for nurses) compared with those taking antidepressant medication who generated 316 extra consultations per 1000 patients.

People taking medication for asthma or COAD generated almost as many extra consultations as those on antidepressants. Whilst only 20% of this is with practice nurses, in absolute terms this means that COAD and asthma combined actually accounted for slightly more work for nurses than people with diabetes or hypertension.

Table 17.6: *Extra* consultations per 1000 patients on the list, 1998

Condition	(A) For doctors	(B) For nurses	(C) Total
Diabetes	14	51	65
Coronary heart disease	56	27	83
Hypertension	80	56	136
Ulcer-healing drugs	131	12	145
Asthma/COAD drugs	248	61	309
Antidepressants	316	16	332

In this study, the total number of consultations per 1000 patients for all reasons was 3151 for doctors and 883 for practice nurses.

Some conclusions

What conclusions could be drawn about how practices deliver care to people with these chronic conditions? And how might practices and PCGs choose to respond to these results in terms of their skill mix and service planning?

From a general practice perspective, the extra activity due to long-term illness is a result of:

the extra consultations associated with the condition

× the number of people with the condition

- Some serious conditions, such as diabetes and CHD, actually constitute a rather small percentage of practice consultations due to their low prevalence in the population. This has implications for practices examining how to respond to Health Improvement Programmes (HImPs). Making improvements in how practices handle people with CHD, for example, is unlikely to cause any big increase in their overall work, though we recognise that any period of change-over to a new approach involves initial extra effort.
- Over the last few years practice nurses have taken on an increasing role in the care of chronic disease. These results indicate that this is most advanced for diabetes where the bulk (77%) of the consultations are now being done by practice nurses. This suggests that when diabetes becomes a HImP priority, strategies for better practice need to be tuned to practice nurse needs rather than to GPs' views.
- A similar but less pronounced effect can be seen with hypertension and CHD. Practices might wish to review how doctors and nurses share the work of CHD and hypertension. Is their current split the right one for them? Or would it make sense to move further down the road of a nurse-led service for these patients too?

- By contrast, people having treatment for asthma or other forms of COAD are much more numerous in the population and generated 8% of all doctor in-surgery consultations. The evidence of this study suggests that only about 20% of the care of these people is currently being undertaken by practice nurses. Is there potential for rationalising the service these people receive, either by using existing consultations more systematically or by moving further to nurse-led clinics for these conditions?

- People taking ulcer-healing drugs, antidepressants or antipsychotics consult a lot. Why are they consulting? Perhaps these are people who are consulting inappropriately or have other unrecognised problems? Are they people who need a longer consultation to talk through what is wrong in greater depth? If doctors can give these people a more effective service then it is likely to have a large effect on their workload as well as improving their patients' health.

- If a person has an ulcer-healing drug, antidepressant or antipsychotic visible on the medication screen, it is probable that they consult fairly frequently. Consultations with such people might be more effective if the clinician is conscious that they could well be a relatively frequent attender.

- The extra consultations generated by people taking antidepressants constituted 10% of all consultations with a doctor in-surgery. How can GPs improve the service to this group? Some might usefully be seen by other mental health professionals, such as counsellors, but the numbers involved mean that GPs will remain the appropriate source of professional help for most of these people. People taking antipsychotics are relatively uncommon but their individual consultation rates were highest of all. Is there a greater role for community psychiatric nurses in their treatment?

- Lack of home visit data for all the practices makes the situation for the care of the very elderly hard to interpret. There was a suggestion, however, for some conditions of a diminishing of the link between chronic illness and extra consultations, even after examining the data from one practice for home visits. Is the care of the very elderly more geared to responding to immediate problems rather than to managing a long-term condition, and is this appropriate?

Further information

Further information can be found in our report:

* *Looking After Long-term Illness: implications for practice consultation rates*, October 1999.

Morbidity rates

Further information about morbidity rates can be found in:

* McCormick A, Fleming D and Charlton J (1959) *Morbidity Statistics from General Practice: fourth national study 1991–1992.* HMSO, London.
* Department of Health (1998) *Key Health Statistics from General Practice, 1996.* ONS, London.
* Colhoun H and Prescott-Clarke P (1996) *Health Survey for England, 1994.* HMSO, London.

Key points

* Patients with long-term illness consulted both GPs and practice nurses in-surgery markedly more than patients of the same age and sex who did not have the illness. This was true for both men and women, more or less for all ages, and in every individual practice that provided data.

- The extra consultations generated were markedly greater *per patient* for the more psychologically-based conditions than for the physical illnesses.
- Ten per cent of all GP consultations were attributable to the extra consultations generated by patients taking anti-depressants, and 8% were due to patients taking medication for asthma/COAD. In contrast, diabetes generated less than 0.5% of GP consultations, and CHD less than 2%.
- The data suggested that over 75% of the care of diabetics was being undertaken by practice nurses, as was 40% of the care of hypertension, 33% for CHD and 20% for asthma/COAD. Care of these four conditions seemed to account for 22% of practice nurse consultations, which represents a large increase since the 1991 NMS.
- Various suggestions are made about the implications of this data for how practices manage long-term illness.

What others have found

Schellevis F, Van de Lisdonk E, Van der Velden J *et al.* (1994) Consultation rates and incidence of inter-current morbidity among patients with chronic disease in general practice. *British Journal of General Practice.* **44**: 259–62.

Patients with diabetes or hypertension in a Dutch general practice had significantly higher consultation rates than age–sex-adjusted controls. Patients with co-morbidity, i.e. more than one of five chosen chronic conditions; consulted more than those with just one. It was not, however, a simple linear association since they tended to bring several problems to the same consultation.

Neville R, McKellican J and Foster J (1988) Heroin users in general practice: ascertainment and features. *BMJ.* **296**: 755–8.

Heroin addicts in Dundee had significantly higher consultation rates than a control group, this difference being entirely accounted for by consultations related to their addiction.

Charlton I, Charlton G, Broomfield J *et al.* (1991) Audit of the effect of a nurse-run asthma clinic on workload and patient morbidity in a general practice. *British Journal of General Practice.* **41**: 227–31.
Introducing a nurse-run asthma clinic led to better quality care of patients with asthma. The increase in nurse consultations was slightly more than the drop in GP consultations for the patients attending the clinic.

Box 17.2:   Do it yourself?

The database used in this study has been developed into a tool-kit that can enable practices to input their own data to benchmark their populations against these results. It is written in Microsoft Access 6 and designed for highly automated input of data from the Front Desk computer appointment system that many Meditel practices have, and of clinical data extracted using Miquest software. It can take appointment and clinical data from other sources but the user will require a greater knowledge of Access. It is available for download from the library section of our website: www.innovate.org.uk

---

18 Are there economies of scale in the employment of administrative and reception staff?

In most fields of activity there are economies of scale as organisations get larger, though this is perhaps less true in service activities than in production. In general practice we might expect that the supporting administrative activities would provide more potential for such economies than the one-to-one contact of the consultation. In particular, since a hypothetical single-handed GP with only 100 patients would still need to employ a receptionist for much of the week, as well as some secretarial and administrative back-up, we intuitively expected some advantages to accrue with greater list size.

Figure 18.1, for 26 Sheffield practices in 1996, demonstrates that they varied greatly in their number of administrative staff hours per 1000 patients – from 25 to 53.

Figures are based on a normal working week and exclude overtime. 'Admin' *included* practice managers, administrators, secretaries, receptionists and computer workers but *excluded* cleaners and staff employed specifically on fundholding tasks, such as fund managers and data entry clerks. Where staff were partly employed for General Medical Services (GMS) work and partly for fundholding, only their GMS hours were included.

No attempt was made to break down the admin category further into, say, receptionists, secretaries, etc. because administrative staff often cross boundaries in what they do, and the same job may be called 'head receptionist' in one practice and 'assistant practice manager' in the next.

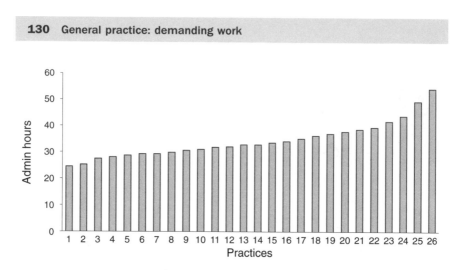

Figure 18.1: Administration hours per 1000 patients.

The issue of role boundaries has wider ramifications. A practice with high admin staff levels may, for instance, have managerial staff who are undertaking work that elsewhere would be done by the partners or practice accountant at a higher cost. The accessibility of a practice may also be an issue in that practices with longer opening hours or more telephone lines may require a higher level of reception staffing. Whether a high level of admin staff is cost-effective, or leads to a better quality service, is for individual practices to judge.

Figure 18.2 plots the relationship between the number of admin

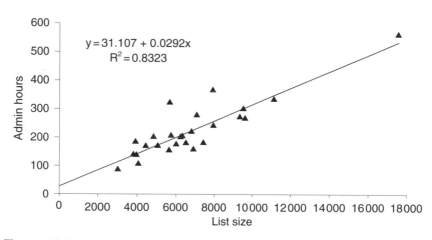

Figure 18.2: Administration hours vs. list size.

hours in each practice and the list size. It attempts to address the issue of whether there are economies of scale in general practice.

The sloping line on Figure 18.2 (the 'regression' line) represents the best-fit relationship between list size and the necessary number of admin hours. It produces an equation which suggests that a practice needs about **31** hours of admin time per week just to get started. This is what economists would call a 'fixed cost', which will weigh more heavily on small practices. After that it needs about another **29** hours of admin time for every extra 1000 patients, regardless of list size. The fact that the data is best fitted by a straight line rather than a curve suggests that there are no other economies, or diseconomies, with increasing list size. The R^2 value of 0.83 means that 83% of the variation in number of admin hours per practice can be accounted for by practice list size.

Practices above the regression line have a higher than average number of admin hours whilst those below it are lower than average. Once again, no judgement is implied as to what is the most cost-effective level of staffing.

Figure 18.3 is similar to the previous one but replaces list size, as a proxy measure of patient demand, by surgery contacts. This is the number of consultations with either a doctor or a practice nurse in the surgery during the year April 1st 1996–March 31st 1997. There

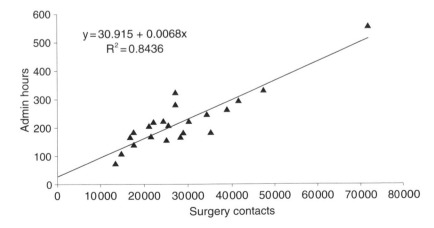

Figure 18.3: Administration hours vs. surgery contacts.

is no clear-cut measure of how patient demand generates workload for admin staff, though it is reasonable to assume that surgery consultations generate more work for receptionists than home visits. For simplicity, therefore, surgery consultations were used as a measure of patient demand.

The relationship found in Figure 18.3 is remarkably similar overall to Figure 18.2 based on list size, suggesting that once again a practice needs about **31** hours of admin time to start up and, after that, a further **6.8** hours for every 1000 surgery consultations per year.

Box 18.1:   Statistician's health warning

Drawing generalisable conclusions from only 26 practices is somewhat risky. A statistician would say that a different set of practices might throw up different results. For instance, removing the single outlying practice with over 17 000 patients increases the initial number of admin hours needed in Figure 18.2 to 46, and reduces the number of extra hours per 1000 patients to 27. Therefore our conclusions should be treated with some caution and should be seen as no more than useful 'rules of thumb'.

Further information

Further information can be found in our report:

* *How Does Our Nursing Administrative Staff Provision Compare With Other Practices in PDC?* November 1997.

Key points

- There was a more than twofold variation in the number of admin hours per 1000 patients amongst 26 Sheffield practices.
- The data suggested that a practice needs about 31 hours per week of administrative staff to get started, but there was no evidence of any further economies of scale in the employment of admin staff in larger practices.
- The data suggested that every extra 1000 patients on the practice list required another 29 hours of admin staff, or alternatively every extra 1000 GP/practice nurse surgery consultations required another 6.8 hours of admin staff.
- Practices might find these figures useful 'rules of thumb' in taking decisions about their administrative staff needs.

Box 18.2: Thinking big?

Our analysis suggests that there is not much scope for economies of scale within a single practice. But what if we change the focus and, in the era of primary care trusts (PCTs), think in terms of services provided across several practices or perhaps even a whole PCT. Recent years have shown the value of such an approach to out-of-hours care. So what about having a single 0845 telephone number to call which would:

- take appointments on computer for all the surgery sites
- use NHS Direct triage and advice as an additional option for patients calling for appointments
- take all telephone requests for repeat prescriptions. This would allow an in-house pharmacist plus doctor with access to computer records to deal with most of the repeat prescription problems before they were sent through to the base surgery

- take all requests for in-hours visits. These could be centrally triaged to filter out those that needed advice only and prioritise those that were urgent/emergencies.

A central organisation could also provide a range of other back-up services which individual practices could opt into or not, such as:

- payroll administration
- IT advice and support
- building management
- bulk purchase of vaccines, clinical and office materials
- personnel
- provision of GP and nurse locums.

Changes such as these would leave admin staff in each practice much freer to concentrate on the personal aspects of dealing with patients. Receptionists, for instance, could be trained to take on new roles in assisting and advising patients to make appropriate use of primary care services, or as medical assistants undertaking phlebotomy and urine testing.

An attractive scenario or a nightmare? Views will vary. We do not doubt for one minute the professional, technical (common IT system) and logistical obstacles to be overcome but neither do we doubt that in some places, some aspects of this scenario will begin to emerge. NHS Direct is not only here to stay but will become more integrated with GP services. At first this will be with GP co-op out-of-hours cover, but in time the logic of its development will suggest that the nurses it employs should be able to directly book patients in to see their GP.

The Internet will also make its contribution. A few practices already give patients their internal practice computer number. They can then log onto the practice's website and book appointments directly using the number as a PIN. Whilst this is clearly a middle-class past-time at present, the imminent arrival of interactive digital TV is likely to provide this opportunity to many more patients and practices.

19 Consultations in general practice: what do they cost?

When we have to decide about shifting services from secondary to primary care, the cost to practices in terms of consultation rates aren't known or included. They are a freebie. They don't cause us any pain. (Health authority manager)

Historically, the price that the NHS or other bodies have paid for GPs' time has been decided largely on the basis of the political bargaining power of the respective players. At the same time, cash-strapped health authorities and hospitals have had an economic incentive to transfer activity to general practice. The resulting work is usually subsumed within the nationally financed budget of General Medical Services, though increasingly GPs have argued for, and sometimes won, extra local payments for specialist work, such as the treatment of drug addicts.

As primary care groups and primary care trusts develop, and primary and secondary care expenditure is increasingly brought under one framework, the potential for cost shifting diminishes. For a PCG/T, or an individual practice, the decision whether to shift the provision of a service from secondary care to general practice requires an accurate understanding of the cost of provision in both locations. Analysis of hospital activity from a health economist perspective is relatively well developed. Less work has been done on the cost of a general practice consultation and there has been debate over the method to use.

We wanted to try and answer the question that a PCG/T board or individual GP might reasonably ask:

'If we were to provide a new service in general practice, or transfer an existing hospital-based service to general practice, what would be the additional consultation costs incurred in providing that service?'

Examples of such a service might be treating drug addicts, running a special clinic for a chronic condition or providing an anticoagulation service. The aim was to produce some cost estimates that could be of practical use to all those within the NHS who have to take decisions about resource use within general practice.

Approach

Measuring the cost of a consultation sounds as though it should be straightforward. In fact, you have to very clear about what it is exactly you are measuring, whose perspective is being adopted, and where and what time period you are concerned about (so as to allow for inflation). There is no single measure of the cost of a consultation with a GP or a practice nurse. Box 19.1 explains this further.

In this study we took the **perspective of a PCG or PCT** as an overseer of resource allocation. We were looking at the **opportunity cost** to a practice in providing the consultation, and we sought to calculate the **marginal cost** of providing an extra daytime surgery consultation or home visit by either a GP or a practice nurse.

Box 19.1: Health economics explained

Are you calculating **average costs or marginal costs?** The average cost to the NHS of providing a GP consultation needs to take into account all expenditure that led up to that consultation. This includes the cost of training the GP, the

---

capital cost of the building and its ongoing running costs, as well as the salary of the GP and any staff involved in supporting the consultation. Such average costs, sometimes excluding long-term training, are usually referred to as **unit costs**, and are what people usually measure in the NHS.

The marginal cost is something different. It is the cost involved in providing *one* more consultation. Normally, capital costs or training costs are irrelevant when considering marginal costs as they do not change with small increases in activity. The fundamental concern in marginal costing is the extra costs generated by that additional consultation.

It is also important to distinguish between **financial cost** as commonly understood, and the economist notion of **opportunity cost**. Undertaking an additional consultation does not necessarily generate any direct financial cost (it would if it led to somebody being paid to work longer). It may instead lead to another piece of general practice work being dropped, or the GP or practice staff having less leisure time. The opportunity cost of the consultation is, strictly speaking, the value of the activity that has been forgone in order to undertake the consultation. In practice, economic studies usually use wages or salaries to represent the opportunity cost of the use of an individual's time.

The perspective adopted is also crucial. A consultation by a practice nurse, for instance, costs the NHS rather more than it costs their GP employer because most of the nurse's salary is reimbursed from NHS funds. From a societal perspective, a complete analysis of costs would also take into account the cost to the patient of the time involved in attending the surgery and the cost to their employer.

Our interest was in the kind of new service that might generate another 50–500 consultations per year in an average practice. This would not be sufficient to require the practice to expand its building, take on an extra partner or purchase new computer equipment. We also assumed that the service took place during normal surgery opening hours. This meant that many items of practice expenditure, such as building costs or computer equipment, would be unchanged and could be excluded from the analysis. It also meant that we were not trying to cost out-of-hours cover.

We also excluded, as others had done, the cost of any prescribed medication or clinical materials used since these will always depend on the type of consultation. We sought a more general costing, based principally on the **time** taken both by the consultation and by all the activities linked to it.

We used data for the **financial year 1997–98** and, wherever possible, for England as a whole. At times this had to be supplemented with local data from Sheffield. However, no attempt was made to develop regional costs, with no account being taken, for instance, of the London weighting for practice staff.

A study that explored the average cost of NHS expenditure on a consultation in 2000, including the costs of medication dispensed, building provision and training of the GP, would come to very different conclusions.

The model used

Any costing of a consultation needs to:

- identify the types of inputs needed to provide the consultation
- determine how much of each input is used
- quantify the cost of the input.

Table 19.1 indicates the methodology used by this study, which is a modified version of that proposed by Hughes (1991). Previous studies have tended to focus on the time spent by GPs (and occasionally nurses) and then add on other 'overheads' in a very

Table 19.1: The model used

Type of input	Measure of input	Value of input
GP: time spent on consultations and other activities linked to the consultation, e.g. phone calls, referral letters, lab tests, repeat scripts, reading mail, clinical discussions	Minutes	Pro rata proportion of gross income from General Medical Services
Practice nurse: time spent on consultations and other activities linked to the consultation, e.g. phone calls, lab tests, clinic administration, mail, computer data entry, clinical discussions	Minutes	Pro rata proportion of gross salary + employer's National Insurance (NI) contribution + pension
Ancillary staff: time spent on reception and administrative tasks related to the consultation, e.g. phone calls, booking appointments, repeat scripts, filing, pulling notes, computer data entry, typing letters, claim forms	Minutes	Pro rata proportion of gross salary + employer's NI contribution + pension
Administrative materials, e.g. telephone calls, postage, photocopying, printing	Quantity	Market prices
Transport costs for home visits	Miles	Market prices

general way. This study sought to identify in greater detail the time spent by GPs and nurses, and to directly include the time spent by ancillary staff.

Direct administrative costs such as phone calls, paper and photocopying charges were included. However, administrative overheads such as telephone and photocopier rental were excluded. Building and other overheads were excluded for the reasons given earlier. Charges for heat and light were also ignored. Data from the accounts of four Sheffield practices indicated that even the *average* heat and light costs of a consultation were only 9p. The extra *marginal* cost of a consultation in a surgery that is already open will be negligible.

Table 19.2: Results from the standard model

		GPs		Practice nurses	
		Surgery consultation	Home visit	Surgery consultation	Home visit
(A)	Face-to-face consultation time (mins)	8.7	25.2	9*	27
(B)	Time spent in linked activity (mins)	3.6	3.6	12.5*	12.5
(C)	Cost per minute	£0.42	£0.42	£0.22	£0.22
(D)	Clinician cost per consultation = (A + B) × C	£5.17	£12.10	£4.73	£8.69
(E)	Ancillary staff time spent in consultation-linked activities	15.8	15.8	15.8	15.8
(F)	Cost per minute	£0.12	£0.12	£0.12	£0.12
(G)	Ancillary staff cost per consultation = E × F	£1.90	£1.90	£1.90	£1.90
(H)	Administrative materials cost	£0.26	£0.26	£0.26	£0.26
(I)	Travel cost		£0.50		£0.50
Total marginal cost per consultation D + G + H + I		£7.32	£14.75	£6.89	£11.35

* Chapter 12 details how for practice nurses the distinction between time spent consulting and consultation-linked activity is a very grey one. Consequently, rather more confidence can be placed in the total time per consultation spent in both activities (A + B = 21.5 minutes) than in the time allotted to the two constituent parts. Fortunately, for the model the cost calculation for practice nurse surgery consultations is based on the combined total A + B.

Table 19.2 presents the results of applying the model using the best available data and assumptions. The cost of a GP in-surgery consultation in this study was estimated at £7.32, that of a practice nurse at £6.89. A GP daytime home visit was estimated to cost £14.75, and a practice nurse home visit £11.35. (**Remember that this is 1997–98 data. To update to 2000, add 10% for inflation.**)

A key aim of the study was to present the methodology, data sources and assumptions made, transparently and in some depth. This enables others to apply the model as times change, or using different, perhaps better, data sources and assumptions. It is not appropriate here to present all those detailed assumptions, but they are available in our report *Consultations in General Practice: what do they cost?*, December 1999.

Principal data sources

Much of the data for this study was available from published national sources:

- Netten A, Dennett J and Knight J (1999) *Unit Costs of Health and Social Care, 1998.* Canterbury Personal Social Services Research Unit.
- *General Medical Practitioners' Workload Survey, 1992–93. Final Analysis* (1994) Joint evidence to the Doctors' and Dentists' Review Body from the Health Departments and the GMSC.
- Department of Health (1999) *Statistics for General Medical Practitioners in England: 1988–1998.* DoH, London.
- The monthly magazine *Medeconomics.*
- Atkin K and Hirst M (1994) *Costing Practice Nurses: implications for primary health care.* Discussion paper 117, Social Policy Research Unit, University of York.

Data on practice staff pay rates was provided by Sheffield Health Authority, since the Department of Health does not collect such data nationally. Occasionally, use needed to be made of our own data, particularly for how practice nurses and administrative staff spend their working week. This included a self-completed week long survey in four practices of what each member of staff was doing every 15 minutes.

Sensitivity analysis

A model is only as good as the data and assumptions on which it is based. The purpose of sensitivity analysis is to focus on those factors that have the greatest impact on the cost estimates, such as GP income or nurse pay, and demonstrate the effect of changing the main assumptions. The results in Table 19.3 indicate the range in which the costs of the different types of consultation will lie.

Analyses 1–4 compare the results when key data is changed, generally by ±25%. This scale of variation is large but occurs in the real world of general practice without being an extreme case. For all four analyses there is evidence that this level of variation encompasses about 90% of general practices.

1 GP income from General Medical Services varies, principally according to the number of patients the GP has on their list. High-income GPs will cost more per consultation than low-income GPs. The average whole-time equivalent English GP in 1997 had 1982 patients. Adding or subtracting 600 patients does not simply raise/lower the GP's income by 30% because not all GMS income is based on list size. Therefore the calculation here assumes that a 30% change in list size leads to a 25% change in income.

2 Similarly, pay rates for practice nurses vary. The average rate for practice nurses in Sheffield in 1997–98 was on the cusp of Whitley Council scales F and G. Table 19.3 shows the effect on consultation cost of a nurse pay rate at the bottom of F and the top of G.

3 The cost of a consultation for a GP who consults in 6.5 minutes

Table 19.3:   Sensitivity analysis

Marginal cost per consultation	GPs		Practice nurses	
	Surgery consultation	Home visit	Surgery consultation	Home visit
1 Low-income GP with 1400 patients	£6.03	£11.73	–	–
1 High-income GP with 2600 patients	£8.61	£17.78	–	–
2 Low-paid nurse – bottom of scale F	–	–	£6.03	£9.77
2 High-paid nurse – top of scale G	–	–	£7.32	£12.14
3 Quick-consulting GP or nurse – 25% faster	£6.02	£12.99	£5.71	£9.84
3 Slow-consulting GP or nurse – 25% slower	£8.62	£16.52	£8.06	£12.85
4 Ancillary staff costs – 25% lower	£6.85	£14.20	£6.41	£10.87
4 Ancillary staff costs – 25% higher	£7.80	£15.23	£7.36	£11.82
5 Low GP income, nurse pay and ancillary staff costs	£5.56	£11.25	£5.55	£9.29
5 High GP income, nurse pay and ancillary staff costs	£9.09	£18.25	£7.79	£12.61
6 Scenario A – extreme high-cost GP and nurse	£10.10	£19.75	£9.14	£14.44
6 Scenario B – extreme low-cost GP and nurse	£4.92	£10.28	£4.52	£7.87
7 Locum GP on BMA rates	£8.31	£11.37	–	–
Sensitivity analysis – extreme range	£4.92–£10.10	£10.28–£19.75	£4.52 – £9.14	£7.87–£14.44
Sensitivity analysis – 90% range	£5.56–£9.09	£11.25–£18.25	£5.55–£8.06	£9.29–£12.85
Central estimate	£7.32	£14.75	£6.89	£11.35

will be less than for one who takes 10.9 minutes. Table 19.3 shows the effect of altering the length of consultation and other linked time for both GPs and nurses by ±25%. (For home visits only, the face-to-face time with the patient was varied by 25%, not the 12 minutes of travel time.)

4   The cost of ancillary staff per consultation can vary for a number of inter-linked reasons, depending on their pay rates, numbers employed, speed of work and the consultation rate of the practice. Here we raised/lowered the overall cost by 25%.

Analyses 1 to 4 are **one-way sensitivity analyses**, in that only one variable is changed at a time. In the real world, changes in one variable affect another. Some changes in costs will tend to cancel each other out. High-income GPs with many patients may well only be able to cope with such high numbers by having short consultation times. Other changes may work in the same direction. A high-earning general practice may pay their nurses on a high scale point and may have unusually high staff costs. Analysis 5 is a **two-way sensitivity analysis**, in that GP or nurse income and ancillary staff costs are allowed to co-vary in the same direction by ±25%.

Analysis 6 presents **extreme scenarios**. Not so extreme as to be ridiculous, but practices that within a PCG/PCT of 20 practices *could* represent the polar ends of the spectrum.

Scenario A is a high-earning practice with a list size of 2600 patients per partner. It has a low annual patient consultation rate of 2.6 surgery consultations with a GP, and the partners have no outside commitments. This allows them, despite the high list size, time for ten-minute consultations and more generally to take 15% longer than the average in their work. Their practice nurses are paid at the top of scale G and take 25% longer than the average to see patients, etc. Their ancillary staff costs are 25% above average, as are their administrative materials and travel costs.

Scenario B is a low-earning practice with a list size of 1400 patients per partner. It has a high annual patient consultation rate of four surgery consultations with a GP, and the partners have a number of outside commitments to supplement their income. This means that, despite the low list size, they have to consult fairly quickly (7.4 minutes) and more generally they take 15% less time than the average in their work. Their practice nurses are paid at the bottom of scale F and take 25% less time than the average to see patients, etc. Their ancillary staff costs are 25% below average, as are their administrative materials and travel costs

Analysis 7 introduces a different kind of scenario. It calculates the cost of a GP consultation if undertaken by a locum doctor. The cost per minute was based on the mid-point of the British Medical Association (BMA) recommended rate in 1997 – £30 per hour in surgery, £8 per daytime home visit. These results suggest that locum cover is more expensive than a GP for surgery consultations, but cheaper for home visits. However, it can be argued that locum doctors consult quicker than a GP (*see* Chapter 12 for evidence).

Discussion

No account has been taken here of the cost of any prescriptions generated. The publication *Unit Costs of Health and Social Care* (Netten *et al.* 1998) estimated that the **average prescription cost per consultation is £17.80.** They calculated this by dividing the cost of prescriptions in general practice by the total number of GP consultations. This figure includes all repeat prescriptions which were assumed to have arisen from initial consultations. Since some repeat prescribing in general practice is effectively initiated by hospital doctors, the £17.80 figure is arguably an overestimate. Clearly, when a new service in general practice is being considered, the costs associated with prescribing can be considerably more than the labour costs, depending on the type of service being provided, and need to be given careful consideration.

Perhaps the most unexpected conclusion of this study is that the difference in marginal consultation cost between GPs and practice nurses was so small. This requires further explanation.

The implicit 'hourly rate' of GPs for GMS work is nearly twice that of practice nurses. Practice nurses, though, have a 'throughput' of patients of only 57% of the rate of GPs when one takes into account the extra work that each does in preparation for, or in follow-up of, the consultation. However, these differences may arise because the two professions have different roles and responsibilities and do different kinds of work.

It may be entirely appropriate that acute medical care takes less time per consultation than the chronic disease management or health promotion that forms a major part of the work of practice nurses. Such work by nurses may require more follow-up beside the face-to-face consultation. It may also be the case that GPs, as the employer, receive more administrative support from their staff than do practice nurses. Ultimately, any study of the cost-effectiveness of GPs versus practice nurses would need to take into account the differing benefits and outcomes for patients of the work of the two professional groups.

Finally, we must stress that we have only looked at the general practice end. Any decision to shift a service from secondary to primary care has to also look at the marginal savings made in the hospital as well as the benefits and costs to the patients in terms of quality of care and outcomes.

Further information

Further information can be found in our report:

* *Consultations in General Practice: what do they cost?* December 1999.

Key points

* There can be no single estimate of the cost of a consultation with a GP or practice nurse. The answer depends on

what exactly one is measuring, where and when, and whose perspective is being adopted.

- Table 19.4 presents our best estimate of the **marginal opportunity** (largely labour) **cost in 1997–98** of GP and practice nurse surgery consultations and home visits. It also presents a range of estimates within which 90% of general practices will lie.
- Increases in GP fees and practice staff wage levels mean that to arrive at the equivalent figures for 2000 one should add on about 10%.
- The small difference in surgery consultation cost between GPs and nurses, despite practice nurses being paid at approximately half the rate of GPs, is because their throughput of patients is only 57% of GPs. This can perhaps be attributed to practice nurses having a different role to GPs, more focused on health promotion and chronic disease management, which encompasses a less intensive style of consultation.
- The costs of a consultation presented here are significantly less than the average cost of the prescriptions it can generate, which have been estimated by others to be £17.80 per consultation if all repeat prescribing is taken into account.

Table 19.4: Summary of marginal costs

		Central estimate	Range
Surgery consultation	GP	£7.32	£5.56–£9.09
	Practice nurse	£6.89	£5.55–£8.06
Daytime home visit	GP	£14.75	£11.26–£18.25
	Practice nurse	£11.35	£9.29–£12.85

What others have found

Studies of the cost of a GP or practice nurse consultation have come to very different conclusions based on very different assumptions, methodologies and perspectives.

Hughes D (1991) Costing consultations in general practice: towards a standardised method. *Family Practice.* **8**: 388–93.
> We took Hughes' proposed method and made some modifications of our own.

Netten A, Dennett J and Knight J (1999) *Unit Costs of Health and Social Care, 1998.* Canterbury Personal Social Services Research Unit.
> This is the most authoritative source of cost estimates in the NHS. Netten *et al.* arrived at a figure of £14 for a GP consultation, but that is based on the average unit cost to the Department of Health, taking into account capital and overhead costs plus the full cost of training a GP, and some administrative costs incurred by the health authority in supporting general practice. Their figure falls to £10 if training costs are omitted. On a similar basis they arrived at £7.29 for the average cost of a practice nurse consultation to the NHS in 1997–98, and £9.84 for a 20-minute home visit.

Graham B and McGregor K (1997) What does a GP consultation cost? *British Journal of General Practice.* **47**: 170–2.
> This review article looked at 11 studies, containing 14 different estimates and using very different methodologies. However, they felt that only four had a sufficiently rigorous methodology, and amongst these the average unit cost (excluding training) of a ten-minute GP consultation at 1995–96 prices was £7.78.

Atkin K and Hirst M (1994) *Costing Practice Nurses: implications for primary health care.* Discussion paper 117, Social Policy Research Unit, University of York.
> Atkin and Hirst looked at average costs, including overheads for practice nurses in 1992–93, and calculated a figure of £22.24 per

hour of patient contact. Applying that figure to the data on nurse activity used in this study, and allowing for nurse pay rises over the period, would give an average cost per consultation of £7.16, and for a home visit of £11.33.

Venning P, Durie A, Roland M *et al.* (2000) Randomised controlled trial: comparing cost-effectiveness of general practitioners and nurse practitioners in primary care. *BMJ.* **320**: 1048–53.
  Venning *et al.* measured the GP/nurse salary costs of about 650 consultations with each, plus the cost of prescriptions, tests, referrals and the cost of return consultations in the following two weeks. Despite their lower salary, nurse costs were only 12.5% lower due to longer consultations, more return consultations and more tests carried out.

Kernick D, Reinhold D and Netten A (2000) What does it cost the patient to see the doctor? *British Journal of General Practice.* **50**: 401–3.
  This article takes a radically different perspective by looking at the cost to the patient of a GP consultation in travel and lost wages. They calculate it at £4.84 if aged over 65 years and £5.45 if aged under 65 years. These figures were less than a third of the costs of attending medical outpatients.

Examples of cost studies of a specific service in general practice

- Koperski M (1992) Systematic care of diabetic patients in one general practice: how much does it cost? *British Journal of General Practice.* **42**: 370–2.
- O'Cathain A, Brazier J, Milner P *et al.* (1992) Cost-effectiveness of minor surgery in one general practice: a prospective comparison with hospital practice. *British Journal of General Practice.* **42**: 13–17.
- Fall M, Walters S, Read D *et al.* (1997) An evaluation of a nurse-led ear care service in primary care: benefits and costs. *British Journal of General Practice.* **47**: 699–703.

- Latimer V, Sassi F, George S *et al.* (2000) Cost analysis of nurse telephone consultation in out-of-hours primary care: evidence from a randomised controlled trial. *BMJ.* **320:** 1053–7.
- Friedli K, King M and Lloyd M (2000) The economics of employing a counsellor in general practice: analysis of data from a randomised controlled trial. *British Journal of General Practice.* **50:** 276–83.

20 Continuity, vocation and the changing nature of GP work

Everyone working in primary care over the last few years has found their work changing. GPs often find this particularly hard to cope with since they usually see themselves as the keystone of the system, and in addition have had to cope with many entirely new roles such as fundholder, manager and PCG board member. This chapter is written entirely from a GP perspective and examines this sense of 'role drift'. It first appeared in the British Journal of General Practice, June 2000.

There is a profound sense of unease abroad amongst general practitioners. We comfort ourselves with familiar excuses – overwork, patient expectations, too much enforced change – but in reality the roots of our unease run deeper. The truth is that for years we have been giving away our core roles: birth takes place in hospitals, death in hospices. Night calls (remember them?) have been taken over for most of us by cooperatives and deputising services – the MacDonalds of the NHS – cheerful, effective places that do not pretend to nourish. Systematic care of chronic illness is done more effectively by nurses and minor illness is triaged away.

Many of these changes have been for good reason: like everyone else we wanted an easier life, and the old ways were variously unacceptable to patients, politicians, partners or ourselves. Yet the result is a hollowing out of the GP's professional role. We have had some splendid new clothes of course – PCG chairs, fundholding, hundreds of academic posts – but underneath we cannot help but wonder what it is that we are about. What is our job description? What do we do that is really worth £50 000 per year?

Whistling in the dark we call up old tunes – continuity of care, personal doctoring, universal accessibility, gatekeeping – but old laurels fade. Patients typically rate continuity of care way below communication, competence and accessibility. And the one kind of continuity that they do want, to be able to see the same doctor about the same problem, is the last thing that we offer.

Such doubts are reinforced by a self-imposed impotence. For entirely understandable reasons the profession, managers and politicians collude to keep many of the most effective new interventions from British patients. Contrast beta-interferon, dona-zepil, Viagra, leucotrienes, Relenza with meningitis C vaccine and statins. All are new and expensive, but in Britain only the life-saving ones have any chance of funding. At each new innovation you can almost hear the academic wheels grinding to find respectable reasons to justify limited use. And with devolved budgets, our relief when they do is as great as our collusion. In this new conspiracy against the laity, quality of life and symptom relief come to be seen as relatively unimportant, and many things that might help us to 'comfort often' are collusively foresworn.

For some, a salaried service offers salvation: let GPs get on with what they are good at (whatever that is) and leave the management to others with better skills. Around 20% of job adverts in the *British Medical Journal* are currently for salaried positions, and for many more the thought of being salaried is becoming a comforting fantasy to fall back on. Yet whilst the new salaried posts are exciting and innovative, it is difficult to see how they can be the salvation of the GP role. It is hard to get the economics of a salaried service to add up – if GPs are no longer going to manage the service, a new layer of managers will be needed to do all those things that previously partners did 'for free'. This will either mean that salaried partners will be paid less or the service will cost more. Furthermore, a large number of salaried posts makes the pool system of reimbursement for self-employed GPs increasingly unstable.

So far, so grim, but what is to be done? First, let's junk the rhetoric. We don't need our comfort blankets about continuity of care any more. People want fast, efficient, courteous service from professionals who are competent, who will discuss fully what can be done and be completely transparent about why sometimes things will not be done. This is not rocket science but while we are perceived to be failing to deliver it, we are dead in the water.

Secondly, the *only* scientific reason for forcing the public to see generalists rather than go direct to specialists is that the predictive value of signs and symptoms is different for low-prevalence populations than for high. This means that generalists are much better at diagnosing normality ('I don't know what's wrong with you but it isn't serious') than specialists, and so it is in the patient's interest to see a generalist first. This is the real reason why the epiphenomenon of gatekeeping works, and it is a truth that needs shouting from the rooftops for it is the only enduring reason to have generalists as the first point of contact.

We also need to be much more open about our manifest conflicts of interest. Caring for individual patients *routinely* conflicts with our role as resource manager, and it is no accident that money is our last taboo. We can talk about sex, death, incest, abuse, complaints and any kind of deviancy with our patients – but we never talk about what things cost. Like all taboos, this one is rooted in shame – shame in our serving two masters whilst pretending to be dedicated solely to patients.

We need to invent new tools for the future. A new procurement system for IT, for example, that ensures stable investment in a few high-quality systems and allows us to junk our current criminally inadequate legacy systems. This has little to do with system specification (as laid out in the RFAs) and everything to with reconstructing the way we set up the market so that PCTs can make sensible investment decisions and suppliers have a stable market. And we need new ways to think about capital. For decades general practice has had the financial equivalent of anorexia. GPs looking in the mirror have seen a well-fed, decently capitalised practice. In reality, primary care has been chronically under-capitalised, starved of investment and unable to mature properly. PCTs give some hope of breaking this cycle: a PFI to buy premises across a whole PCT would solve several problems at a stroke. The release of current capital back to GPs would create enormous goodwill; the PCT would get the flexibility to plan new buildings; and most important of all it would create a whole new raft of people and mechanisms that could bring financial imagination and planning to primary care.

All this will help us to do the job better but does not speak to the void that is growing at the heart of practice. To fill this we need to recognise that meaning and the search for meaning are central to doctoring and to healing. Patients come to us asking, Why me? Why now? Why this disease? What next? Am I going to die? Here at the heart of our medicine there can be no guidelines, no easy answers. For we do not create the patient's meaning but merely witness, reflect, inform their enduring search. And nor is the search limited to that arbitrary set of others known as 'patients'. The enduring search is ours too. The mantle of doctor, taken so easily, cloaks our own search for meanings, the dilemmas and wounds of our own unfolding lives and lifelong fascination with disease and death.

To speak of these things, to place this as central to what we do, seems to invite ridicule from the inner cynic. Yet silence does a disservice too. Thirty years ago, in *A Fortunate Man*, John Berger described John Sassall, a GP, as fortunate:

> *Sassall is nevertheless a man doing what he wants . . . Sometimes the pursuit involves strain and disappointment, but in itself it is his unique source of satisfaction. Like anybody who believes that his work justifies his life, Sassall – by our society's miserable standards – is a fortunate man.*

Today we have come to believe that our work only has to justify our paycheck, and in consequence we rattle with hollow dissatisfaction at ourselves. Technique, organisation, science – all are necessary but not sufficient to move beyond this sense of emptiness. The human search for meaning lies at the heart of medicine and at the core of vocation. Sometimes, if we are fortunate, such work goes beyond the mundane and we find ourselves participating in a small instance of the sacred.

21 Concluding thoughts

This chapter summarises some of the key conclusions of the book and concludes with some thoughts about how practice might respond to pressure to increase accessibility to patients.

Key conclusions

- GP contact rates in large urban areas are some 20–30% higher than the national average reported in the Fourth National Morbidity Survey in 1991/2. This will partly be due to higher morbidity in urban areas, but arguably the NMS underestimated contact rates.
- Contact rates are not rising. GP in-surgery consultation rates are static, whilst home visiting rates are declining, in part due to the advent of out-of-hours cooperatives. GP consultations have, however, become more complex and the amount of paperwork has increased.
- The consultation and visit workload for GPs is higher in the winter, but the seasonal difference is less than might have been expected.
- Practice nurse contact rates rose sharply in the early 1990s, in large part due to a major increase in the numbers of practice nurses employed. The expansion in nurse numbers has now largely stopped and contact rates are static. The only seasonal pattern in their work is the autumn bulge of influenza vaccinations.

- Within any given practice there is no consistent connection between one kind of work and another. For example, high numbers of GP consultations do not consistently lead to low or high numbers of hospital referrals, more or fewer out-of-hours calls, or greater or lesser numbers of consultations with practice nurses. Similarly, undertaking many home visits during the day is not linked to more (or less) out-of-hours contacts.
- Consultation rates for GPs vary widely between practices and there is hardly any detectable rhyme or reason to this variation. Both our data and the wider literature support the conclusion that practice profile, list size, number of partners, distance from hospital or gender of doctor – none of these accounts for the large differences that may be found between adjacent practices. Only deprivation to some modest degree causes a consistent increase in consultation rates.
- The large differences between practices in nurse consultation rates can be largely explained by one variable – the number of nursing hours per week. Nurse consultation rates bear no relation to any measure of need or demand.
- Exploring these differences is valuable because it illuminates practice and philosophy, and highlights where people can learn from each other.

We entitled this book *Demanding Work*. In one sense this is a misnomer. For practice nurses, the number of consultations they undertake is overwhelmingly rooted in practice decisions about how many nurse appointments to *supply*. Even for GPs, what they experience as an incessant demand is in fact a complex interaction of the decisions they take about how many appointments to supply and the decisions patients take about what to demand. We suggest that the decisions about supply are the principal governors of GP workload, and reflect deeper decisions about the kind and quality of service GPs wish to provide.

The complex interaction between supply and demand now takes place in the context of a government committed to 'modernisation' of the service. For general practice, modernisation includes reducing the number of days that patients have to wait to see a GP, with the aim of 90% of patients who want it being seen within one day. Can your average general practice meet this target? Our work (*see* Chapter 11) would suggest that, as currently structured, almost all of today's GP appointment systems will fail.

A cynical response would be to return to largely drop-in surgeries. Instead of waiting days, patients would have to sit for (only) hours to see a GP. The target would be met but neither patients, GPs nor government would be happy.

An alternative response is to argue, as the BMA does, for more doctors – cut the waiting lists by significantly increasing the supply. They have a point. The average full-time British GP has to care for about 1900 patients – significantly more than in most developed countries. But in the British context it will take many years to achieve a significant increase in supply. Indeed, the supply of GPs in the next decade will be hard-pressed to keep pace with the numbers retiring or leaving the profession.

For a practice seriously wanting to cut its waiting times, what could it do? There is no magic bullet, rather a range of options that could help:

- **Do the patients need to see a GP?** The role of practice nursing expanded considerably during the early 1990s, particularly in the areas of health promotion and chronic disease management. However, as we have shown in Chapter 17, there is considerable scope for further expansion even in this area. The use of practice nurses, or nurse practitioners, in triage roles for acute minor illness is still relatively uncommon within general practice, but destined we suspect for a major expansion.

  This would require more practice nurses, and the finance to pay for them, and is another variant of the BMA's 'more resources' argument. Nurses are quicker to train than GPs, and there is much more scope for luring trained people back into the profession, though we would warn against those who think this is a cheap option (*see* Chapter 19).

- **Does it have to be a nurse?** Whilst nurses will make the largest impact, other professions could play a role in freeing up GP time. We've already referred to the role of counsellors or therapists with frequent attenders. Greater potential, in our view, lies with community pharmacists. We do not mean another government advertisement for people to seek advice from their fast-disappearing local community pharmacy. We think the future lies more with community pharmacists employed directly within primary care. (*See*, for instance, Morris S and Warner B (2000) Can dinosaurs learn to dance? *British Journal of General Practice.* **50:** 254–5.)

- **Does the patient have to be *seen*?** In this electronic age, why shouldn't a significant number of consultations be conducted on-line? As electronic communication moves away from the expensive computer to the cheaper mobile phone or interactive TV, this means of communication will become available to most of the population. But before leaping into the 21st century, how about embracing that classic 20th-century form of communication, the ordinary telephone. At various points in the book we have referred to the potential for phone communication to replace home visits *and* surgery consultations.

- **Does the patient need an *appointment*?** GPs prefer the predictable workload of appointment-based surgeries. In general, it does lead to a better service. We think most patients, most of the time, prefer it that way too. But it may be the case that some general practices have gone too far down that road. In our view, a good appointments system has to make a significant allowance for same-day appointments/drop-ins for acute illness.

Will all this allow practices to see 90% of patients within one day? Probably not, partly because, as we've argued, an increase in supply will to some extent lead to an increase in demand.

It is easy for the government to set populist targets. Achieving them is *demanding work* and requires the long-term goodwill and collaboration of all those who work in general practice. Every suggestion in this book for change in general practice is presented, and we hope taken, in that spirit.

Appendix 1
Contact rates from the Fourth National Morbidity Study 1991/2

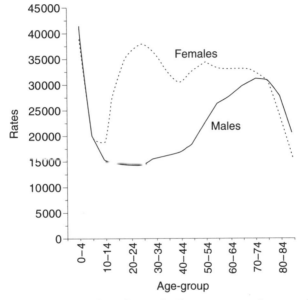

Figure A1.1: Contacts with a doctor in the surgery, rates per 10 000 person years at risk.

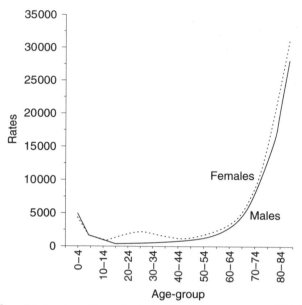

Figure A1.2: Contacts with a doctor at home, rates per 10 000 person years at risk.

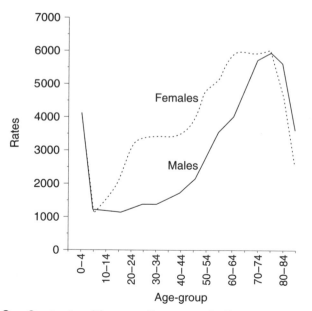

Figure A1.3: Contacts with a practice nurse in the surgery, rates per 10 000 person years at risk.

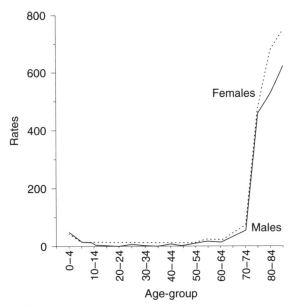

Figure A1.4:   Contacts with a practice nurse at home, rates per 10 000 person years at risk.

Source: McCormick, Fleming and Charlton (1995). Reproduced by kind permission of the authors.

Appendix 2
Guide to activity data collection

GP surgery consultations

Definition

A face-to-face consultation between a GP and a patient on the practice list, within the practice building, resulting in patient note entry.

Source of data

Use a source which gives accurate numbers with the least extra work needed to extract the data. Totalling daily numbers of filled appointments from the appointment book, if you run one, and adding in any extras may be a good way.

Include:

- multi-consultations – where the GP treats and makes notes on another person who attends with the person who had the appointment. A consultation should be recorded for each person so treated, although only one appointment may have been made
- patients passed from another clinician who makes notes as well as the GP. A consultation should be recorded for each clinician although only one appointment may have been made.

Exclude:

- DNAs

- patients who left before consultation, i.e. those who did turn up, checked in but left (e.g. through frustration) before seeing a GP.

Practice nurse surgery consultations

Definition

A face-to-face consultation between the nurse and a patient on the practice list, within the practice building, resulting in patient note entry.

Source of data

Use a source which gives accurate numbers with the least extra work needed to extract the data. Totalling daily numbers of filled appointments from the appointment book, if you run one, and adding in any extras may be a good way.

Include:

- multi-consultations – where the nurse treats and makes notes on another person who attends with the person who had the appointment. A consultation should be recorded for each person so treated, although only one appointment may have been made
- patients passed from another clinician who makes notes as well as the nurse. A consultation should be recorded for each clinician although only one appointment may have been made.

Exclude:

- DNAs
- patients who left before consultation, i.e. those who turned up, checked in but left (e.g. through frustration) before seeing a nurse.

Home visits by practice nurse

Definition

A contact between a practice nurse and a patient on the practice list, outside the practice building, resulting in patient note entry.

Source of data

Often a visit book or nurse diary will be the best source for these figures, but look out for the following.

Include:

- consultations with more than one member of a family. (This should be counted as a consultation per person.)

Exclude:

- patients who were not in when the nurse called 'on spec'. (Will it be clear from the diary that the visits did not in fact take place?)

GP daytime home visits

Definition

A home visit:

- to a patient on the practice list (including temporary residents)
- that *is not* a health authority-claimable night visit
- that *is not* made by the deputising/GP co-op service.

Source of data

Normally this would be some form of visit book.

GP night visits

Definition

A home visit:

- to a patient on the practice list (including temporary residents)
- that *is* a health authority-claimable night visit
- that *is not* made by the deputising/GP co-op service.

Source of data

Normally this would be the system of claiming the night visiting fee from the health authority.

Deputising/co-op service night visits

Definition

A home visit:

- to a patient on the practice list (including temporary residents)
- that *is* a health authority-claimable night visit
- that *is* made by a deputising/GP co-op service.

Source of data

Invoices from the deputising/GP co-op service to the practice.

Deputising/co-op service non-night visits

Definition

A home visit:

- to a patient on the practice list (including temporary residents)
- that *is not* a health authority-claimable night visit
- that *is* made by a deputising/GP co-op service.

Source of data

Invoices from the deputising/GP co-op service to the practice.

Deputising/co-op service night 'surgery consultations'

Definition

A visit made by a patient on the practice list to a deputising service surgery or primary care centre between 10 p.m. and 6 a.m.

Source of data

Invoices from the deputising/GP co-op service to the practice.

Deputising/co-op service 'surgery consultations' made at other times

Definition

A visit made by a patient on the practice list to a deputising service surgery or primary care centre outside 10 p.m. to 6 a.m.

Source of data

Invoices from the deputising/GP co-op service to the practice.

Deputising/co-op service 'advice calls'

Definition

An advice call made to a patient on the practice list (including temporary residents) by the deputising/GP co-op service.

Source of data

Invoices from the deputising/GP co-op service to the practice.

Index